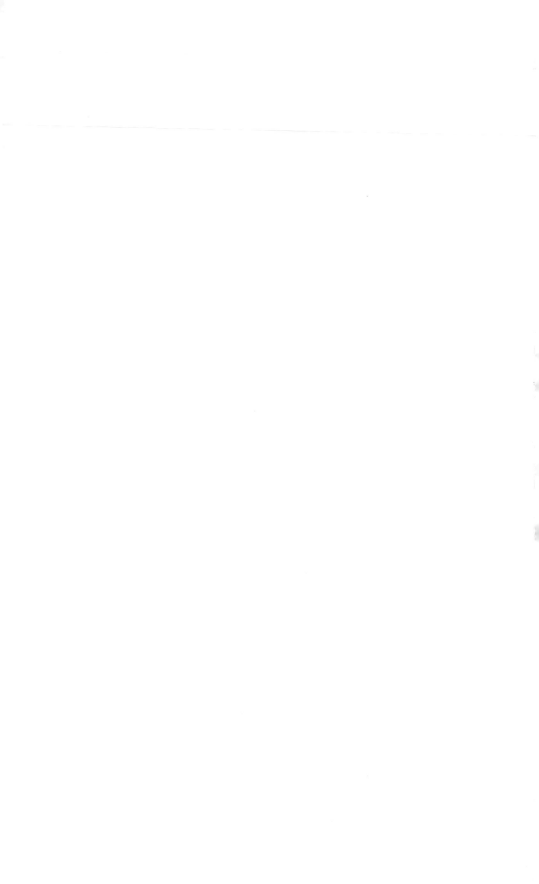

Acne

Recent Titles in
Q&A Health Guides

Smoking: Your Questions Answered
Stacy Mintzer Herlihy

Teen Stress: Your Questions Answered
Nicole Neda Zamanzadeh and Tamara D. Afifi

Grief and Loss: Your Questions Answered
Louis Kuykendall Jr.

Healthy Friendships: Your Questions Answered
Lauren Holleb

Trauma and Resilience: Your Questions Answered
Keith A. Young

Vegetarian and Vegan Diets: Your Questions Answered
Alice C. Richer

Yoga: Your Questions Answered
Anjali A. Sarkar

Teen Pregnancy: Your Questions Answered
Paul Quinn

Sexual Harassment: Your Questions Answered
Justine J. Reel

Sports Injuries: Your Questions Answered
James H. Johnson

Essential Oils: Your Questions Answered
Randi Minetor

Hormones: Your Questions Answered
Tish Davidson

Marijuana: Your Questions Answered
Aharon W. Zorea

Exercise: Your Questions Answered
Justine J. Reel

ACNE

Your Questions Answered

Shayan Waseh

Q&A Health Guides

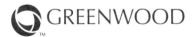

An Imprint of ABC-CLIO, LLC
Santa Barbara, California • Denver, Colorado

Library of Congress Cataloging-in-Publication Data

Names: Waseh, Shayan, author.
Title: Acne : your questions answered / Shayan Waseh.
Description: Santa Barbara, California : Greenwood An Imprint of ABC-CLIO, LLC, [2023] | Series: Q&A Health Guides | Includes bibliographical references and index.
Identifiers: LCCN 2022026200 | ISBN 9781440879685 (hardcover) | ISBN 9781440879692 (ebook)
Subjects: LCSH: Acne—Popular works. | Acne—Miscellanea.
Classification: LCC RL131 .W37 2023 | DDC 616.5/3—dc23/eng/20220606
LC record available at https://lccn.loc.gov/2022026200

ISBN: 978-1-4408-7968-5 (print)
         978-1-4408-7969-2 (ebook)

27 26 25 24 23   1 2 3 4 5

This book is also available as an eBook.

Greenwood
An Imprint of ABC-CLIO, LLC

ABC-CLIO, LLC
147 Castilian Drive
Santa Barbara, California 93117
www.abc-clio.com

This book is printed on acid-free paper ∞

Manufactured in the United States of America

Contents

Series Foreword	ix
Acknowledgments	xi
Introduction	xiii
Guide to Health Literacy	xv
Common Misconceptions about Acne	xxiii
Questions and Answers	1
The Basics	3
1. What is acne? Are there different types?	3
2. How common is acne?	5
3. Is acne contagious?	6
4. How does acne affect the skin?	8
5. Where does acne appear?	10
6. What is the spectrum of acne severity?	12
7. Why does acne tend to happen in adolescence?	14
8. Does acne also occur outside of adolescence?	15
9. How does acne differ in skin of color?	17
10. What is the difference between acne and rosacea?	19
11. What other conditions can mimic acne?	21

The Causes of Acne   25

    12. Why does acne happen?   25
    13. How do hormones affect acne?   27
    14. What medical conditions can cause acne?   29
    15. Can stress affect acne?   31
    16. How does weight gain affect acne?   32
    17. Do alcohol and smoking influence acne?   34
    18. How does diet affect acne?   35
    19. Can wearing makeup cause acne?   38
    20. Is acne caused by poor hygiene?   39
    21. Is there a genetic component to acne?   41
    22. How does pregnancy influence acne?   42
    23. What medications can cause or worsen acne?   44
    24. What are some red flags that indicate a
        more serious form of acne?   46

Living with Acne   49

    25. How does acne impact self-image?   49
    26. Can having acne lead to depression?   51
    27. Is it okay to pick at acne bumps?   53
    28. Does anything help make acne less itchy?   55
    29. Can you wear makeup with acne?   56
    30. How can I change my skin-care routine to
        help with acne?   58
    31. What other lifestyle modifications can help with acne?   60
    32. What support resources are available for
        people with acne?   62

Acne Treatments   65

    33. When does acne need to be treated by a doctor?   65
    34. What types of doctors are trained to treat acne?   67
    35. What is benzoyl peroxide? How does it help acne?   69
    36. Can antibiotics help with treating acne?   71
    37. How do topical retinoids help with acne?   72
    38. What is isotretinoin (Accutane)?   74
    39. What is the iPLEDGE program?   76
    40. How is hormonal acne treated differently than
        other types of acne?   78
    41. Can light therapy be helpful in treating acne?   80
    42. What cosmetic treatments can help with acne?   82

43. Does alternative medicine offer any effective
     treatments for acne? 83
44. What are the common side effects of acne treatment? 85
45. How long does it typically take to effectively treat acne? 86
46. Is treating acne expensive? 88

Managing the Skin after Acne 91

47. Can acne reoccur? 91
48. Does acne have any long-term impact on the skin? 92
49. Why can skin become lighter or darker after
     acne goes away? 94
50. What causes acne scarring? 95
51. How common are acne scars? 97
52. Is there a way to minimize the chance of
     developing acne scars? 98
53. Are acne scars permanent? 100
54. What treatments are available for acne scarring? 101

Case Studies 103

Glossary 117

Directory of Resources 121

Index 123

Series Foreword

All of us have questions about our health. Is this normal? Should I be doing something differently? Whom should I talk to about my concerns? And our modern world is full of answers. Thanks to the Internet, there's a wealth of information at our fingertips, from forums where people can share their personal experiences to Wikipedia articles to the full text of medical studies. But finding the right information can be an intimidating and difficult task—some sources are written at too high a level, others have been oversimplified, while still others are heavily biased or simply inaccurate.

Q&A Health Guides address the needs of readers who want accurate, concise answers to their health questions, authored by reputable and objective experts, and written in clear and easy-to-understand language. This series focuses on the topics that matter most to young adult readers, including various aspects of physical and emotional well-being as well as other components of a healthy lifestyle. These guides will also serve as a valuable tool for parents, school counselors, and others who may need to answer teens' health questions.

All books in the series follow the same format to make finding information quick and easy. Each volume begins with an essay on health literacy and why it is so important when it comes to gathering and evaluating health information. Next, the top five myths and misconceptions that surround the topic are dispelled. The heart of each guide is a collection of questions and answers, organized thematically. A selection of five case studies provides real-world examples to illuminate key concepts. Rounding out each volume are a directory of resources, glossary, and index.

It is our hope that the books in this series will not only provide valuable information but will also help guide readers toward a lifetime of healthy decision making.

Acknowledgments

My deepest thanks go to my loved ones who have supported me through every stage of my journey in medicine and service to humanity. To my parents, for their selfless love and sacrifices. To my remarkable wife, for her endless support and companionship. To my precious children, for their unending inspiration and wonder. I am overwhelmed by the gift of love that you have each ceaselessly shared with me, and I would never have been able to journey this far without each of you.

Thank you as well to all of the friends, colleagues, and mentors that have illuminated my path throughout my career. Particularly, great thanks are owed to the late Dr. Loghmanee, who sparked my passion in medicine and vivified so many others through his dedication to service and humanity. In addition, thank you to the Department of Dermatology at Thomas Jefferson University for introducing me to the world of dermatology and to the Department of Dermatology at Temple University for training me to be a dermatologist empowered to help others. Also, thank you greatly to ABC-CLIO and Maxine Taylor for this opportunity to share my knowledge and experiences regarding acne with others who may be interested in the topic.

Finally, thank you to those of you who are reading this. Your thirst for knowledge and desire to read are responsible for the movement of the world and the advancement of humanity. I have spent countless hours in both my childhood and my adulthood reading in library nooks and school study rooms, and those who read and love reading and learning are deeply inspiring.

Introduction

Acne is unique among all medical conditions. Are there any other medical conditions that affect almost every single person in the world at some point in their life? Are there any other medical conditions that are so visible and that so commonly affect people who are at the most sensitive period of their lives?

I hope that this book adequately addresses the most special and fascinating condition that we refer to as acne. It is a condition that is so common, and yet it can be so hard to find a comprehensive and accurate source of knowledge on the topic. The Internet can be a clash of conflicting sources, and adolescents, teenagers, and young adults can have a hard time knowing where to turn. Therefore, I hope that this book can serve as a source of accurate and insightful knowledge regarding acne.

From the basics of what acne is, what causes acne, and how acne is treated, this book hopes to tackle the most common questions that dermatologists and other physicians are asked regarding acne. During a dermatology appointment, there are typically only a few minutes available to diagnose acne, prescribe a treatment, and educate a patient regarding his or her acne. This book is a collection of all the knowledge that I wish I could share with each of my acne patients. In fact, I wish that every person in the world could know all of the information that is in this book. Acne is so common that it is almost less like a medical condition and more like a commonly shared human experience.

I hope that this book will illuminate the topic of acne for those who are interested. Some may have acne themselves and be searching for knowledge regarding the topic. Others might have an interest in medicine and caring for others. Still others may be interested in knowledge for knowledge's sake. Whatever your reason for reading, I believe that you will find this book an appropriate and informative guide, and I hope that you enjoy reading it as much as I enjoyed the experience of writing it.

Guide to Health Literacy

On her 13th birthday, Samantha was diagnosed with type 2 diabetes. She consulted her mom and her aunt, both of whom also have type 2 diabetes, and decided to go with their strategy of managing diabetes by taking insulin. As a result of participating in an after-school program at her middle school that focused on health literacy, she learned that she can help manage the level of glucose in her bloodstream by counting her carbohydrate intake, following a diabetic diet, and exercising regularly. But, what exactly should she do? How does she keep track of her carbohydrate intake? What is a diabetic diet? How long should she exercise and what type of exercise should she do? Samantha is a visual learner, so she turned to her favorite source of media, YouTube, to answer these questions. She found videos from individuals around the world sharing their experiences and tips, doctors (or at least people who have "Dr." in their YouTube channel names), government agencies such as the National Institutes of Health, and even video clips from cat lovers who have cats with diabetes. With guidance from the librarian and the health and science teachers at her school, she assessed the credibility of the information in these videos and even compared their suggestions to some of the print resources that she was able to find at her school library. Now, she knows exactly how to count her carbohydrate level, how to prepare and follow a diabetic diet, and how much (and what) exercise is needed daily. She intends to share her findings with her mom and her aunt, and now she wants to create a chart that summarizes what she has learned that she can share with her doctor.

Samantha's experience is not unique. She represents a shift in our society; an individual no longer views himself or herself as a passive recipient of medical care but as an active mediator of his or her own health. However, in this era when any individual can post his or her opinions and experiences with a particular health condition online with just a few clicks or publish a memoir, it is vital that people know how to assess the credibility of health information. Gone are the days when "publishing" health information required intense vetting. The health information landscape is highly saturated, and people have innumerable sources where they can find information about practically any health topic. The sources (whether print, online, or a person) that an individual consults for health information are crucial because the accuracy and trustworthiness of the information can potentially affect his or her overall health. The ability to find, select, assess, and use health information constitutes a type of literacy—health literacy—that everyone must possess.

THE DEFINITION AND PHASES OF HEALTH LITERACY

One of the most popular definitions for health literacy comes from Ratzan and Parker (2000), who describe health literacy as "the degree to which individuals have the capacity to obtain, process, and understand basic health information and services needed to make appropriate health decisions." Recent research has extrapolated health literacy into health literacy bits, further shedding light on the multiple phases and literacy practices that are embedded within the multifaceted concept of health literacy. Although this research has focused primarily on online health information seeking, these health literacy bits are needed to successfully navigate both print and online sources. There are six phases of health information seeking: (1) Information Need Identification and Question Formulation, (2) Information Search, (3) Information Comprehension, (4) Information Assessment, (5) Information Management, and (6) Information Use.

The first phase is the *information need identification and question formulation phase*. In this phase, one needs to be able to develop and refine a range of questions to frame one's search and understand relevant health terms. In the second phase, *information search*, one has to possess appropriate searching skills, such as using proper keywords and correct spelling in search terms, especially when using search engines and databases. It is also crucial to understand how search engines work (i.e., how search results are derived, what the order of the search results means, how to use the snippets that are provided in the search results list to select websites, and how to determine which listings are ads on a search engine results page). One also has to limit reliance on surface characteristics, such as the design of a website or a book (a website or book that appears to have a lot of information or looks aesthetically pleasant does not necessarily mean it has good information) and language used (a website or book that utilizes jargon, the keywords that one used to conduct the search, or the word "information" does not necessarily indicate it will have good information). The next phase is *information comprehension*, whereby one needs to have the ability to read, comprehend, and recall the information (including textual, numerical, and visual content) one has located from the books and/or online resources.

To assess the credibility of health information (*information assessment* phase), one needs to be able to evaluate information for accuracy, evaluate how current the information is (e.g., when a website was last updated or when a book was published), and evaluate the creators of the source—for example, examine site sponsors or type of sites (.com, .gov, .edu, or .org) or the author of a book (practicing doctor, a celebrity doctor, a patient of a specific disease, etc.) to determine the believability of the person/organization providing the information. Such credibility perceptions tend to become generalized, so they must be frequently reexamined (e.g., the belief that a specific news agency always has credible health information needs continuous vetting). One also needs to evaluate the credibility of the medium (e.g., television, Internet, radio, social media, and book) and evaluate—not just accept without questioning—others' claims regarding the validity of a site, book, or other specific source of information. At this stage, one has to "make sense of information gathered from diverse sources by identifying misconceptions, main and supporting ideas, conflicting information, point of view, and biases" (American Association of School Librarians [AASL], 2009, p. 13) and conclude which sources/information are valid and accurate by using conscious strategies rather than simply using intuitive judgments or "rules of thumb." This phase is the most challenging segment of health information seeking and serves as a determinant of success (or lack thereof) in the information-seeking process. The following section on Sources of Health Information further explains this phase.

The fifth phase is *information management*, whereby one has to organize information that has been gathered in some manner to ensure easy retrieval and use in the future. The last phase is *information use*, in which one will synthesize information found across various resources, draw conclusions, and locate the answer to his or her original question and/or the content that fulfills the information need. This phase also often involves implementation, such as using the information to solve a health problem; make health-related decisions; identify and engage in behaviors that will help a person to avoid health risks; share the health information found with family members and friends who may benefit from it; and advocate more broadly for personal, family, or community health.

THE IMPORTANCE OF HEALTH LITERACY

The conception of health has moved from a passive view (someone is either well or ill) to one that is more active and process based (someone is working toward preventing or managing disease). Hence, the dominant focus has shifted from doctors and treatments to patients and prevention, resulting in the need to strengthen our ability and confidence (as patients and consumers of health care) to look for, assess, understand, manage, share, adapt, and use health-related information. An individual's health literacy level has been found to predict his or her health status better than age, race, educational attainment, employment status, and income level (National Network of Libraries of Medicine, 2013). Greater health literacy also enables individuals to better communicate with health care providers such as doctors, nutritionists, and therapists, as they can pose more relevant, informed, and useful questions to health care providers. Another added advantage of greater health literacy is better information-seeking skills, not only for health but also in other domains, such as completing assignments for school.

SOURCES OF HEALTH INFORMATION: THE GOOD, THE BAD, AND THE IN-BETWEEN

For generations, doctors, nurses, nutritionists, health coaches, and other health professionals have been the trusted sources of health information. Additionally, researchers have found that young adults, when they have health-related questions, typically turn to a family member who has had firsthand experience with a health condition because of their family member's close proximity and because of their past experience with, and trust in, this individual. Expertise should be a core consideration when consulting a person, website, or book for health information. The credentials and background of the person or author and conflicting interests of the author (and his or her organization) must be checked and validated to ensure the likely credibility of the health information they are conveying. While books often have implied credibility because of the peer-review process involved, self-publishing has challenged this credibility, so qualifications of book authors should also be verified. When it comes to health information, currency of the source must also be examined. When examining health information/studies presented, pay attention to the exhaustiveness of research methods utilized to offer recommendations or conclusions. Small and nondiverse sample size is often—but not always—an indication of reduced credibility. Studies that confuse correlation with causation is another potential issue to watch for. Information seekers must also pay attention to the sponsors of the research studies. For example, if a study is sponsored by manufacturers of drug Y and the study recommends that drug Y is the best treatment to manage or cure a disease, this may indicate a lack of objectivity on the part of the researchers.

The Internet is rapidly becoming one of the main sources of health information. Online forums, news agencies, personal blogs, social media sites, pharmacy sites, and celebrity "doctors" are all offering medical and health information targeted to various types of people in regard to all types of diseases and symptoms. There are professional journalists, citizen journalists, hoaxers, and people paid to write fake health news on various sites that may appear to have a legitimate domain name and may even have authors who claim to have professional credentials, such as an MD. All these sites *may* offer useful information or information that appears to be useful and relevant; however, much of the information may be debatable and may fall into gray areas that require readers to discern credibility, reliability, and biases.

While broad recognition and acceptance of certain media, institutions, and people often serve as the most popular determining factors to assess credibility of health information among young people, keep in mind that there are legitimate Internet sites, databases, and books that publish health information and serve as sources of health information for doctors, other health sites, and members of the public. For example, MedlinePlus (https://medlineplus.gov) has trusted sources on over 975 diseases and conditions and presents the information in easy-to-understand language.

The chart here presents factors to consider when assessing credibility of health information. However, keep in mind that these factors function only as a guide and require continuous updating to keep abreast with the changes in the landscape of health information, information sources, and technologies.

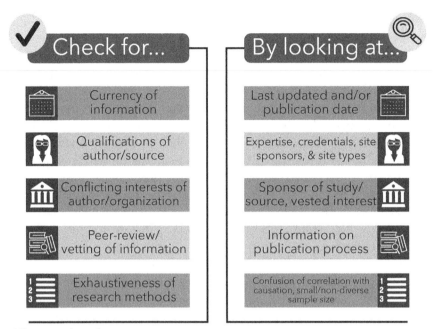

All images from flaticon.com

The chart can serve as a guide; however, approaching a librarian about how one can go about assessing the credibility of both print and online health information is far more effective than using generic checklist-type tools. While librarians are not health experts, they can apply and teach patrons strategies to determine the credibility of health information.

With the prevalence of fake sites and fake resources that appear to be legitimate, it is important to use the following health information assessment tips to verify health information that one has obtained (St. Jean et al., 2015, p. 151):

- **Don't assume you are right**: Even when you feel very sure about an answer, keep in mind that the answer may not be correct, and it is important to conduct (further) searches to validate the information.
- **Don't assume you are wrong**: You may actually have correct information, even if the information you encounter does not match—that is, you may be right and the resources that you have found may contain false information.
- **Take an open approach**: Maintain a critical stance by not including your preexisting beliefs as keywords (or letting them influence your choice of keywords) in a search, as this may influence what it is possible to find out.

- **Verify, verify, and verify**: Information found, especially on the Internet, needs to be validated, no matter how the information appears on the site (i.e., regardless of the appearance of the site or the quantity of information that is included).

Health literacy comes with experience navigating health information. Professional sources of health information, such as doctors, health care providers, and health databases, are still the best, but one also has the power to search for health information and then verify it by consulting with these trusted sources and by using the health information assessment tips and guide shared previously.

Mega Subramaniam, PhD
Associate Professor, College of Information Studies,
University of Maryland

REFERENCES AND FURTHER READING

American Association of School Librarians (AASL). (2009). *Standards for the 21st-century learner in action.* Chicago, IL: American Association of School Librarians.

Hilligoss, B., & Rieh, S.-Y. (2008). Developing a unifying framework of credibility assessment: Construct, heuristics, and interaction in context. *Information Processing & Management, 44*(4), 1467–1484.

Kuhlthau, C. C. (1988). Developing a model of the library search process: Cognitive and affective aspects. *Reference Quarterly, 28*(2), 232–242.

National Network of Libraries of Medicine (NNLM). (2013). Health literacy. Bethesda, MD: National Network of Libraries of Medicine. Retrieved from nnlm.gov/outreach/consumer/hlthlit.html

Ratzan, S. C., & Parker, R. M. (2000). Introduction. In C. R. Selden, M. Zorn, S. C. Ratzan, & R. M. Parker (Eds.), *National Library of Medicine current bibliographies in medicine: Health literacy.* NLM Pub. No. CBM 2000–1. Bethesda, MD: National Institutes of Health, U.S. Department of Health and Human Services.

St. Jean, B., Taylor, N. G., Kodama, C., & Subramaniam, M. (February 2017). Assessing the health information source perceptions of tweens using card-sorting exercises. *Journal of Information Science.* Retrieved from http://journals.sagepub.com/doi/abs/10.1177/0165551516687728

St. Jean, B., Subramaniam, M., Taylor, N. G., Follman, R., Kodama, C., & Casciotti, D. (2015). The influence of positive hypothesis testing on youths' online health-related information seeking. *New Library World, 116*(3/4), 136–154.

Subramaniam, M., St. Jean, B., Taylor, N. G., Kodama, C., Follman, R., & Casciotti, D. (2015). Bit by bit: Using design-based research to improve the health literacy of adolescents. *JMIR Research Protocols*, 4(2), paper e62. Retrieved from http://www.ncbi.nlm.nih.gov/pmc /articles/PMC4464334/

Valenza, J. (2016, November 26). Truth, truthiness, and triangulation: A news literacy toolkit for a "post-truth" world [Web log]. Retrieved from http://blogs.slj.com/neverendingsearch/2016/11/26/truth-truthiness -triangulation-and-the-librarian-way-a-news-literacy-toolkit-for-a-post -truth-world/

Common Misconceptions
about Acne

1. ACNE IS MORE OF AN ANNOYANCE THAN
A SERIOUS MEDICAL CONDITION

Acne is so common that it can be easy to mistakenly think that acne is not a serious medical condition. While some people are not bothered by mild, infrequent acne symptoms, many people do experience discomfort or even embarrassment from their acne. For these people, acne is a serious medical condition that deserves to be treated with the use of safe and effective medications. Importantly, even mild acne can be serious when it disturbs a person's sense of well-being and health, and acne does not have to be extensive or severe to be worth treating. As acne usually occurs on visible parts of the skin, such as the face, it can have an unusually significant impact on the happiness of people who suffer from the condition. To learn more about the serious impact that acne can have on physical and mental well-being, see questions 25 and 26.

2. EVERYBODY EXPERIENCES ACNE IN THE SAME WAY

Despite how common acne is, there is a tremendous amount of variation in how acne affects individuals. While some people might have mild acne that does not bother them, other people can suffer from extensive acne that is life changing. Even in situations where two people have similar amounts of acne, the psychological and emotional impact that the acne has can be different between them. So, although most people experience acne at some point in their lives, no one experiences acne in the same way, and it is important to be mindful of the impact that acne can have on people. To read more about the different forms of acne, see questions 1, 4, 5, and 6.

3. ACNE ONLY AFFECTS ADOLESCENTS AND TEENAGERS

It is true that acne is most common among adolescents and teenagers, especially because the hormonal changes associated with puberty significantly contribute to developing acne. At the same time, however, acne is a skin condition that can affect people of all ages, genders, races, and ethnicities. In fact, there are forms of acne that can affect newborns, children, adults, and even those in their eighties and nineties. Therefore, while acne does primarily impact adolescents and teenagers, it can affect a much broader group of people than most people realize. This topic is addressed in much greater detail in questions 7 and 8.

4. ACNE TREATMENT WORKS QUICKLY AND CAN CURE ACNE WITHIN DAYS

Thankfully, acne is a very treatable skin condition for the vast majority of individuals. In fact, most people can experience complete or near complete improvement of their acne with basic medical treatment. However, treatments for acne often take several weeks to begin to work on the skin and improve acne bumps. In fact, many people actually experience worsening of their acne during the first few days after starting acne treatments. Therefore, the misconception that acne medications will work immediately can be very disheartening for people who start medical treatment for their acne and do not see quick results. To learn more about the way that acne medications work in treating acne bumps, see questions 35, 36, 37, and 38.

5. SCARRING FROM ACNE IS PERMANENT AND CANNOT BE TREATED

One of the most serious outcomes from acne is scarring, especially on sensitive and visible parts of the skin such as the face. This is a big problem because scarring from acne does not heal on its own without treatment and can lead to embarrassment and self-consciousness. So, it is true that acne scarring is permanent, but it is a misconception that there are no treatments for acne scarring. In fact, there are multiple different ways of treating acne scars in the modern era, including the use of lasers, needles, and certain resurfacing medications and treatments. Therefore, while acne scarring can be permanent when left untreated, a variety of treatment options exist for those who suffer from acne scarring. To learn more about the treatment options for acne scars, please refer to questions 53 and 54.

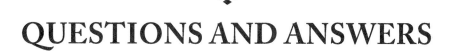

QUESTIONS AND ANSWERS

The Basics

1. What is acne? Are there different types?

Acne is one of the most common skin problems in the United States and the world. Almost everyone experiences acne at some point in their life. While there are different kinds of acne, all acne involves bumps on the skin. These bumps, which are called *papules* by doctors, are caused by dead skin cells and natural skin oils filling up and clogging hair follicles. This is especially common in areas of the body where the skin has a lot of oil glands, like the face, the upper chest, and the back.

When the hair follicle becomes completely blocked off with oils and dead skin cells, this results in a whitehead. When the clogged hair follicles are only partly closed off and still exposed to air, the natural skin oils inside the blockage can become darkened, resulting in blackheads. When the skin has whiteheads and blackheads, this is typically called *classic acne*.

However, both whiteheads and blackheads can get irritated and inflamed and become pimples. When this happens, there is usually a lot of redness, which is another sign of inflammation. If pimples are not treated, they can grow into nodules or cysts and may even result in permanent scarring, which is why treating acne early is so important. If acne has a lot of redness, pimples, nodules, or cysts, it is often labeled as *inflammatory acne* rather than classic acne. Inflammatory acne is often treated with additional medications that work to reduce inflammation in the skin.

There are a lot of other factors that contribute to acne in addition to the clogging of hair follicles and inflammation. Genetics, hormone levels, bacteria, diet, and skin hygiene are all important and can lead to acne or worsen preexisting acne. Most people have multiple different triggers for their acne rather than one single cause, so it is important to treat acne from several angles.

There are also different types of acne beyond the classic and inflammatory forms. *Neonatal acne* is acne in newborn babies that is caused by the mother's hormones affecting the baby shortly after birth. This type of acne typically goes away on its own after a few weeks or months following delivery. It is usually mild and is not treated with medications.

Childhood acne is a type of acne that affects young children and can have a variety of different causes. Sometimes, it is caused by early puberty, but it can also be caused by tumors that release extra hormones into the body, though this is rare. Therefore, children with childhood acne typically get blood tests to make sure they do not have any serious cause for their acne.

Hormonal acne is a type of acne that is caused by extra levels of hormones, such as testosterone, in the body. These hormones can cause acne by increasing the amount of natural skin oils in hair follicles. Hormonal acne typically affects teenage and adult women. Hormonal acne is also typically worse during the menstrual cycle because of the rising levels of hormones during that time. It is often treated with the same medications as classic acne, with the addition of medications that help to normalize the hormones in the body.

Although all of these different forms of acne cause dead skin cells and natural skin oils to clog the hair follicles, the best way to manage each type of acne and the best treatment for each form of acne is different.

While some forms of mild acne can get better with lifestyle changes, acne usually needs to be treated with topical medications that are placed on the surface of the skin. These medications include creams, gels, lotions, and sprays, which work in different ways. Some medications exfoliate the skin, some increase the turnover of cells in the skin, and some target bacteria that live on the skin and contribute to acne. In many people, these medications are enough to significantly improve skin quality and clear acne bumps.

However, when topical medications are not enough, stronger oral medications are used. Some of these oral medications are just stronger versions of the same topical medications used for acne, while other oral medications work in unique ways, such as by affecting the balance of hormones or reducing bacterial activity throughout the entire body. The use of oral medications for the treatment of acne is usually overseen by a general physician or a specialized dermatologist who is trained to monitor effectiveness and manage potential side effects.

Although acne is usually considered a "benign" disease that does not cause people to become seriously ill, it can still be a significant source of distress that decreases self-esteem and increases the risk of mental health issues such as depression and anxiety. The mental health impact of acne is especially large because acne most commonly occurs during puberty and adolescence, when individuals are forming their self-identity and are sensitive to changes in their skin and their general appearance.

Although modern medicine is getting better at treating acne, it continues to be a common and bothersome medical condition for most of the world. Therefore, understanding and being able to treat acne is an important part of promoting international health and well-being on a physical, mental, and emotional level.

2. How common is acne?

Acne is a skin condition that affects almost every person in the world in some form and at some point in their lifetime. Over 600 million people worldwide are affected by acne, making it one of the top ten most common diseases internationally.

In the United States alone, over 50 million people are affected by acne. This is enough to make acne the most common skin condition that affects Americans each year.

Since acne can affect people at any age, about 90% of people report experiencing acne at some point during their lifetime. However, acne most commonly begins in puberty and adolescence and continues throughout young adulthood. Approximately, 85% of people between the ages of twelve and twenty-four go through at least a mild form of acne, while up to 20% of people who get acne suffer from moderate or severe forms of the condition that can seriously impact their quality of life.

Interestingly, getting acne as an adult has become more frequent in recent years, with up to 15% of adult women having acne into their thirties and forties. While the rate of adult acne in men is lower than in women, 1%–5% of adult men still suffer from acne into adulthood. In these adult males, the face and upper chest are usually the most affected skin areas.

In up to 1% of men and 5% of women, acne can continue into later adulthood, including beyond the forties. In these older individuals, acne can be associated with problems in hormone levels or the presence of other medical conditions that contribute to developing acne. Many times, however, there is no clear cause for the acne, and this can make it hard to treat the acne effectively.

Interestingly, recent research has found that acne is much more common in industrialized countries, like those in North America and Europe, than in the nonindustrialized regions of the world. One medical study looked at how common acne is in the Kitavan Islanders of Papua New Guinea and the Aché hunter-gatherers from Paraguay. The study compared the rate of acne in these nonindustrialized populations to that of the United States and found that the rate of acne was much lower among the nonindustrialized groups. This is an interesting finding that has been repeated by multiple other research studies that have made similar comparisons. These research findings could help support the view that hormonal balance, diet, and environment significantly contribute to how common acne is in the modern world.

However, even though there are huge differences in the rate of acne between industrialized and nonindustrialized countries, acne still remains an internationally important disease. The burden of acne on people around the world is very high. In the United States alone, the cost of treating acne and the working time lost due to acne are over a billion dollars every year. Other countries in the world experience a similar problem, highlighting that acne is an important worldwide skin disease.

Society as a whole is becoming more aware of the emotional and psychological impact that acne has on people. Unfortunately, getting access to medical care for acne is still a challenge. In fact, even though over 90% of people suffer from acne at some point in their life, less than 10% of these individuals seek out medical treatment from a dermatologist for their acne. As one of the most common skin diseases in the world, there is a lot more than can be done to get people access to early and effective treatment for their acne.

3. Is acne contagious?

There is a common misconception that acne is contagious. This frequently shared myth often revolves around the claim that sharing skin-care products or having direct skin contact with someone who has acne can cause acne to be transmitted from one person to the other. Thankfully, this is completely false. Acne is never transmitted from one person to another, and there has never been a documented case of contagious acne in history.

However, this myth has continued to exist, and it has caused a significant amount of confusion and even fear. A large part of why the notion that acne might be contagious still exists can be attributed to the fact that bacteria are thought to contribute to the development of acne.

Bacteria and viruses are typically responsible for most contagious diseases. Skin infections, pneumonias, and sexually transmitted diseases can all be caused by bacteria or viruses, and they can be highly contagious, especially to young and old people and those who have weaker immune systems. Since bacteria are responsible for many contagious diseases, it is understandable why some people believe acne might be contagious. However, this belief has long been proven wrong by medical science.

Most importantly, the bacteria that is involved in contributing to acne already lives on the skin of nearly every human being on the planet. This bacterium is known as *Cutibacterium acnes*, or C. *acnes* for short, and it is referred to as a commensal organism. Commensals are organisms that live on or inside of another creature without harming or benefiting them. For example, C. *acnes* lives on the skin of most human beings, and under normal conditions, it would never be noticeable. The bacterium is able to survive through consuming the natural oils of the skin, but it does not cause disease or harm the skin in any way. In fact, it has been estimated that approximately 1.5 trillion bacteria live on the skin, and most of them never impact the skin in a noticeable or negative way.

One of the major issues in acne is that the body produces too many natural skin oils and is not able to get rid of these oils appropriately. This can cause the amount of C. *acnes* bacteria on the skin to grow too large, which can then cause inflammation and make acne worse. Therefore, skin contact between individuals or the sharing of skin-care products does not cause acne because almost everyone already has C. *acnes* living on their skin. In reality, it is each individual's skin environment, the amount of natural oil production, and a variety of other factors that determine whether the individual develops acne. These are ultimately not contagious factors but, rather, unique to each individual.

Importantly, there are a variety of other factors that might make it seem like acne is a contagious disease, even though it is not. Acne is more common in specific age groups, like adolescents, teenagers, and young adults. People in these age groups are more likely to mingle with one another and share a variety of items, including skin-care products and clothing. Therefore, it can seem like these interactions are causing acne to be transmitted between individuals when there are multiple people in a group that develop acne around the same time, but the real culprit is solely that they are all at the most common age for developing acne.

Sharing things like skin-care products, clothing, and towels can sometimes make acne worse, but this effect is not because acne is contagious. If someone uses a makeup brush that has already been extensively used or dries their face with an already dirty towel, they can apply dirt and oils onto their facial skin and clog their skin pores, making acne worse. So, although someone in this situation might believe they "caught" acne from another person, the true contributing factor was the use of already dirtied items.

While the myth that acne is contagious might seem like harmless confusion, it can actually cause a great deal of harm. In those who have acne, it can be embarrassing or even shameful to feel like they are suffering from a contagious disease that they can give to others. These individuals may feel blamed by others and can become afraid and even withdraw from friends and family due to their fears.

In addition, believing that acne is exclusively caused by a contagious bacterium can result in people feeling helpless to treat their acne, and this can cause long delays in getting appropriate medical treatment. In fact, most people can have complete or significant improvement of their acne with simple treatment, and delaying such treatment can cause scarring and other poor cosmetic outcomes. Therefore, it is important to address the myth that acne is a contagious disease and to help promote the understanding that acne is a complex skin condition caused by a variety of factors unique to each individual.

4. How does acne affect the skin?

Acne affects the skin in a number of different ways. To understand how acne affects the skin, it is important to understand the structure of skin and the way that the skin functions normally.

Most of the body's skin surface contains hair follicles. These hair follicles are the small pores on the surface of the skin that hair grows out of. These hair follicles are found on almost every part of the body, except the palms of the hands and the soles of the feet.

In addition to growing hair, hair follicles are attached to tiny microscopic glands known as sebaceous glands. Sebaceous glands make sebum, which is the scientific name for the natural oils of the skin. Therefore, these sebaceous glands can also be called the oil-producing glands of the body.

Once the sebaceous glands produce sebum, they empty the sebum, or natural skin oils, into the hair follicle, where it can travel to the surface of the skin and serve as the natural lubrication of the skin and hair.

These natural oils protect the skin against friction and act as an extra barrier to the outside world, protecting the skin from becoming dry, getting infected by bacteria and other microbes, and being exposed to allergens.

The process of sebum production into the skin's hair follicles is a continuous process that happens every day. In addition, the skin itself is always undergoing change and turnover. In normal skin, individual skin cells grow, mature, and eventually die in a complete life cycle of approximately three weeks. The dying skin cells are slowly pushed toward the surface of the skin and are eventually shed from the body as new skin cells are generated and mature. When these dead skin cells and debris are shed from the body, they fall to the outside world, becoming a form of dust.

In acne, however, these dead skin cells are not correctly shed from the body; instead, they can start to back up and clog the hair follicles and the associated sebaceous glands. This blockage eventually causes natural oils in the hair follicle to build up to abnormally high levels. Bacteria that live on the skin are able to feed on the surplus of these oils, which leads to too many bacteria on the skin, which then leads to inflammation that can make acne significantly worse.

C. acnes, which was formerly known as *Propionibacterium acnes*, is thought to be one of the primary bacteria responsible in this process. This bacterium is part of the normal skin of almost every person on earth and does not typically cause any health problems in healthy adults. However, since it lives off the fatty acids that make up the sebum of the skin, it can easily multiply in number and become overgrown from the extra supply of oil seen in acne. Once the bacteria overgrow, they release chemicals called enzymes that can break down both the fatty acids from sebum and the proteins that the skin uses to keep itself organized and healthy. This breakdown of the normal skin and the sebum can cause inflammation and many of the other features associated with moderate to severe acne.

While these steps that cause acne are shared by individuals who get acne, acne itself can manifest on the skin in many different ways. This is why the symptoms of acne on the skin can vary from blackheads and whiteheads to pus-filled pimples or even nodules and cysts.

In acne's simplest form, blackheads and whiteheads are just areas where pores have become clogged with excess oils, bacteria, and dead skin cells. Blackheads result when these clogged pores are partially open to the environment, resulting in oxidation of the oils in the pore, which turns them black in color. The color of blackheads is not a result of pores becoming clogged with dirt or other dark-colored material, as is commonly incorrectly thought.

On the other hand, whiteheads are the same clogged pores, but they are completely closed off from the environment, which prevents oxidation and keeps the clogged pore contents white in color. Importantly, both of these skin findings of acne, blackheads and whiteheads, lack the irritation and inflammation that causes the pimples, nodules, and cysts that are seen in severe acne.

As previously mentioned, once the hair follicle is clogged and there is an extra amount of sebum, the extra growth of the *C. acnes* bacterium can cause a lot of inflammation to occur. This inflammation causes redness in the skin around the clogged pore and can cause immune cells known as neutrophils to come to the area. The collection of these neutrophils in the skin appears as white pus, and this form of inflammation results in the typical red pimples that are associated with acne.

If these pimples continue to worsen, they eventually form small pus-filled nodules. These nodules are deeper and larger than pimples and can feel like hard knots underneath the skin. This is because nodules do not affect just the top of the skin but also the deeper layers of the skin where the skin's blood vessels and connective tissue are. If left untreated, in some individuals, these small nodules can progress to larger nodules and even cysts, which can leave significant scarring that is permanent unless treated. These cysts are large pockets of pus that have grown into the deep layers of the skin, and they can be extremely red and tender to the touch.

Understanding the roles that hair follicles, sebaceous glands, bacterial overgrowth, and inflammation play in acne allows for a better understanding of how and why acne looks like it does with the presence of whiteheads, blackheads, pimples, nodules, and cysts. Although the complete picture of how acne affects the skin is still being worked out, these factors are thought to be the major drivers of acne in most individuals.

5. Where does acne appear?

Although the blackheads, whiteheads, pimples, nodules, and cysts of acne might look similar between individuals, the locations where they happen and the level of severity can be very different. In fact, when acne occurs on specific parts of the body, it can help to reveal significant clues regarding the cause of the acne and the best way to treat it.

Generally, because problems in skin oil production are a big cause of acne, the bumps of acne are most commonly found on the areas of the skin with the most oil glands. The areas that have a lot of oil glands are the face, neck, chest, and back. Unsurprisingly, these are the areas where acne tends to occur most frequently in most people.

Overall, the face is the most commonly affected area for acne. Unfortunately, it is also one of the most visible and prominent areas of the body and has a lot of social significance. That is why even mild acne can cause significant distress and concern in individuals who are affected by it. Interestingly, the specific location of acne bumps on the face can be a clue as to the cause of the underlying acne and point to the most appropriate treatment.

For example, acne that is mostly caused by high hormone levels, particularly in women, typically affects the skin around the jaw and the sides of the cheeks. In this type of acne, treatment of the abnormally high hormone levels, usually by reducing the level of testosterone, can result in a significant improvement. Additionally, sometimes oral contraceptive medications that contain hormones can help to regulate and normalize the levels of testosterone and estrogen in the body, improving the acne.

In addition, acne frequently develops on areas of the face that are covered or put under pressure on a regular basis. For example, people who sleep with their face on their pillow may develop acne on their cheeks and forehead more frequently than those who do not. Individuals who frequently wear a mask may develop acne on areas of the nose, upper check, and jawline, where the mask sits. Additionally, those who frequently place their hands on their face while working at a desk or while lying down may develop acne of the forehead, cheeks, jaw, and other areas that they regularly touch. In all these situations, the covering of the skin likely causes sebum and dead skin cells to build up on top of the skin surface and in the hair follicle, which causes the hair follicle to become clogged and acne bumps to form. In these situations, reducing the number of contributing factors, such as stomach sleeping or face touching, is an important part of improving the acne.

Beyond the face, acne most commonly affects the upper back, upper chest, lower back, shoulders, arms, and neck. In people with acne on areas other than their face, approximately 50% have acne on their upper back, 30% have acne on the upper chest, 20% have acne on the lower back, 15% have acne on the shoulders and arms, and less than 10% have acne on the neck. Obviously, a meaningful number of people have acne in multiple locations, which can be distressing and challenging.

Although these locations are typically more hidden than the face, acne in these areas can still be a significant source of distress and low self-esteem to all individuals. That is why acne in those areas is still treated with medications, and a variety of shampoos, body washes, creams, and serums have been created for the treatment of acne in these areas.

Also, while it is still relatively common for acne to affect the chest and back, these locations can sometimes be a clue for less common causes of acne. For example, hormone imbalances, such as excess testosterone, especially in men, can cause acne that primarily affects the chest and back without causing acne on the face. This is most commonly seen in young men who use testosterone therapy for the treatment of other medical conditions or who inappropriately use anabolic steroids for muscle building or athletics. In these situations, the acne of the body tends to be widespread and severe. When appropriate, stopping the use of these medications can lead to the acne completely resolving within weeks to months. Further, stopping the use of anabolic steroids or testosterone for reasons other than the treatment of medical conditions is important in people with this type of acne because the use of anabolic steroids is associated with a lot of significant side effects. These serious side effects include liver damage, kidney damage, cardiovascular disease, infertility, and even early death.

Although the location of where acne occurs can be a clue to the underlying cause of the acne, there are some common practices that are not founded on any evidence or science. Acne face mapping is a commonly seen practice that attempts to pinpoint the cause of acne based on the exact location of the face that the acne bumps appear. While there is some truth to this, particularly in acne that is distributed along the skin of the jaw in hormonal acne, acne face mapping attempts to attribute acne to causes such as constipation, pollution, emotions, and other reasons that do not appear likely cause acne to occur in specific parts of the face.

6. What is the spectrum of acne severity?

Although acne is a condition that impacts most individuals at some point in their life, the impact that it can have on the skin is unique to each person that it affects. Therefore, it is important to understand the many forms that acne can take and the wide range of differences that acne can have between individuals on a physical and emotional level. Acne can range from being a mere inconvenience at its most mild to being a debilitating problem in the most severe forms.

Most acne shares the common feature of having bumps on the skin, but the appearance of these bumps can vary significantly. In the mildest forms of acne, these bumps can be the same color as the surrounding skin, and they can be small and difficult to see without looking closely. As acne severity increases, these bumps may change colors, becoming light red, dark red, or even purple, as inflammation and skin damage increases. Additionally, the size of the bumps may increase while they become deeper and more cystic. In severe cases, these bumps can grow together to form cysts and tracts underneath the skin, causing permanent damage. These cysts and tracts are filled with fluid that may be released when they burst as a result of movement or touching.

The amount of skin that is impacted can also vary significantly between individuals. In the majority of people, the skin of the face is the only affected site. Acne in these individuals can impact the cheeks, jawline, nose, eyebrow ridge, and forehead. However, acne can become more extensive and grow to involve the neck, shoulders, chest, back, and torso. While most people's acne affects just 5%–10% of their skin, in severe cases, a majority of the body's skin surface can be affected. In these more extensive forms of acne, the disease tends to be more inflamed and can leave permanent scarring behind.

Importantly, acne can also be labeled differently based on its severity. Although the labels given to different types of acne are not an exact linear spectrum, these various labels can be helpful in classifying how severe an acne is and comparing the different forms of the disease.

For example, when commonplace acne becomes more severe than typically seen and starts to develop into nodules and cysts, this can be labeled as *nodulocystic acne*. In cases where nodulocystic acne gets even worse and becomes disfiguring, the acne is sometimes given the label *acne conglobata*. This form of acne mostly affects young men and leaves significant permanent scarring. When acne becomes even worse than this, causing inflammation in the entire body, it can be labeled as *acne fulminans*. This form of acne can cause high fevers, joint pain, weight loss, spleen and liver swelling, and redness throughout the whole body. This form of acne typically affects young men who are going through puberty, and it requires immediate attention and treatment with medications.

The severity of acne can also differ greatly in regard to how it affects people on a social, mental, and emotional level. In many people with the mildest forms of acne, the condition does not cause any distress and does not affect their appearance, self-esteem, or life in any meaningful way. In individuals with more severe forms of acne, even small areas of acne in highly visible areas of the skin, like the face, can be bothersome and uncomfortable. In the most severe forms of acne, people can be drastically impacted; they become self-conscious and sometimes even develop lifelong mental health issues, such as depression and anxiety. Although acne typically impacts people more as it becomes more severe in appearance, any amount of acne can cause distress in an individual.

7. Why does acne tend to happen in adolescence?

Although acne can affect people of any age, the vast majority of people with acne are adolescents and teenagers. This age group, between the ages of approximately eleven and nineteen, is the most common age group for acne. In fact, studies have shown that somewhere between 85%–90% of people between the ages of eleven and thirty will suffer from acne at some point during that age period.

Most cases of adolescent acne last for about five to ten years without treatment and eventually fade away on their own during the early twenties. However, about one in three adolescents or teenagers will experience a moderate to severe form of acne that may last longer and leave behind scarring.

There are a number of reasons why acne tends to affect adolescents and teenagers more than any other age group. The largest reason, by far, is due to the levels of hormones in the body. During adolescence, the human body goes through the process of puberty, where sex hormones such as testosterone and estrogen increase significantly in males and females, respectively.

In males, the increased level of testosterone in the body during puberty causes height to increase, body and pubic hair to grow, the voice to deepen, muscle mass to develop, and the penis and testicles to increase in size. In females, increased levels of estrogen and progesterone signal the body to begin the process of ovulation and to undergo other physical changes, including the growth of body hair, enlargement of the breasts, and an increase in body fat levels. While testosterone is the primary sexual development hormone in males, as estrogen is for females, testosterone and estrogen both play an important role in both males and females, and the body requires a precise balance of both of these hormones to grow appropriately.

Importantly, these sex-specific hormones also play a large role in influencing the skin health and development of both males and females. Sex hormones signal the oil-producing glands of the skin to increase in size during puberty and begin secreting more of the natural skin oils that are known as sebum. While this process during puberty will eventually result in the oil-producing glands of the skin reaching their adult size and function at the end of young adulthood, the process itself can be disorganized and sometimes not function well during puberty.

This imperfect function can result in extra sebum production, the clogging of hair follicles, and the overgrowth of bacteria that feed on the skin's sebum. These are all contributing factors to the development of acne, and they are the major reasons why acne is so commonly seen in adolescents and teenagers who are undergoing puberty and physical development. The biologic changes happening in the body during puberty create the perfect environment for the development of acne. However, as the final changes of puberty begin to finish in the late teenage years and the early twenties, the body's intense hormonal changes begin to level off and reach a stable balance, allowing most cases of acne to slowly get better and disappear on their own.

Of note, females continue to experience regular changes in the balance of hormone levels in their body, particularly around their period or menstrual cycle. This continuous cycling of hormone levels in the body means that many women suffer from mild to moderate acne around the time of their menstrual period, even into their twenties and thirties. In these individuals, medications like certain forms of birth control and other hormone-blocking medications can help in regulating hormone levels and treating acne.

Although acne primarily affects adolescents, the treatment of acne in all people through the use of facial cleansers, topical antibiotics, and other medications can be extremely effective. While adolescent and teenage acne will often go away on its own over the course of five to ten years, medical treatment can cause acne to get better within weeks and months. Additionally, treating acne can prevent the more severe forms of acne that affect teenagers and prevent the formation of permanent acne scars on the skin. Therefore, while acne is a common skin condition that affects the vast majority of adolescents, it is both treatable and curable in almost all cases.

8. Does acne also occur outside of adolescence?

While the vast majority of acne affects adolescents and teenagers, it still can affect people of all ages. In fact, the proportion of older adults with acne has been slowly increasing over the past few decades. It is unclear why acne is becoming more common in the older age groups, but it is a trend that impacts many lives.

Additionally, special forms of acne can affect newborns, infants, and young children prior to puberty and adolescence. After adolescence, acne may continue to be a persistent problem for some people, and new cases of acne can happen to anyone at any age. In rare cases, new acne has been seen in people who are seventy or eighty years old. However, in most of these extreme cases, there are underlying hormone or other medical conditions that contribute to causing the acne.

Interestingly, newborns can develop a form of acne referred to as *neonatal acne*. The term *neonatal* refers to the period immediately following birth, so neonatal acne is a form of acne that usually starts in newborn babies within two to three weeks of birth and can continue until the baby is up to six months old. This form of acne is actually very common in newborns, with almost 40% of newborns developing some amount of neonatal acne.

These newborns develop small acne bumps on their faces as a result of extra levels of their mother's hormones staying in their body after birth. These elevated hormone levels cause acne to appear, and as the baby gets older and the mother's hormones start to leave the baby's body, the neonatal acne slowly resolves and disappears. Also, because the skin of newborn babies is still developing after birth, they are very sensitive to the impact of hormones and the outside world. Thankfully, this form of acne does not need any medical treatment and never results in scars or permanent skin changes.

Acne can also occur in children slightly older than newborns. This form of acne is referred to as *infantile acne* because it affects infants between the ages of approximately six weeks to one year. This form of acne is more similar to classic acne and can result in whiteheads, blackheads, red bumps, and permanent scarring if it becomes severe and is not appropriately treated. In this age group, the cause of infantile acne is not as well understood as neonatal acne. However, it is believed that there may be genetic differences in hormone production levels during the infant age period that might be partially responsible. Importantly, however, acne in this age group is rare and should be evaluated by a doctor to examine for other potential causes.

In older children who have not yet reached puberty, acne is typically related to increased hormone levels from testosterone and other male sex hormones. It is important to evaluate why these children have elevated hormone levels in their body at their age because it can be due to hormonal diseases, medication side effects, or even tumors that produce hormones.

One example of a tumor that can cause high testosterone levels in children is a testicular tumor that causes abnormal growth of the testicle. The testicles are a major source of testosterone, and overgrowth of a testicle can result in the creation of very high levels of testosterone in the body. In children with this form of tumor, puberty-like changes are experienced at an unusually early age, including rapid growth, the development of body hair, and the presence of severe acne. Importantly, these children often require surgery to remove the testicular tumor before it spreads. While most childhood acne affects newborns and infants without major concern, acne affecting older children under the age of puberty is concerning and requires medical workup.

While adolescence is the most classic time period for acne, it can also affect older adults who have long been done with puberty. In some people, acne from puberty can persist into their twenties and thirties. In others, they may have never experienced acne during puberty but are experiencing it for the first time during their twenties and thirties. In this age group, as in all forms of older adult acne, women are more commonly impacted than men.

Interestingly, the presence of acne in older age groups, from the twenties all the way up to fifty and older, has been increasing over the past few years and decades. In adults fifty and older, approximately 15% of women and 7% of men are still affected by acne. Therefore, acne is increasingly being considered a disease that impacts all ages rather than just adolescents.

In most people above the age of twenty, the presence of acne is still related to the same factors that cause acne during adolescence: hormones, excess oil production, bacterial overgrowth on the skin, and inflammation. However, since acne becomes less common as age increases, acne should be evaluated more seriously in older people. In a small minority of older people with acne, other medical conditions, such as medication side effects or polycystic ovarian syndrome (PCOS), can be contributing to the development of acne. In these cases, treating both the acne as well as the underlying medical condition is essential.

9. How does acne differ in skin of color?

Acne affects people of all skin colors. However, the impact that it has on different skin tones can vary significantly. In fact, acne can look and act quite differently in darker skin types than it does in lighter skin types. Therefore, while two people with different skin types might have the same amount of acne, the way that it affects each person's skin can be very different.

To understand the variation of skin tones in human skin, the Fitzpatrick skin type system is a useful tool. This tool, also known as the

Fitzpatrick scale, is the most common way used by doctors for describing and classifying the color of human skin. This is important because many skin conditions, including acne, can look and act differently in skin of color as compared to lighter skin tones. Being able to easily and reliably categorize skin tone in an objective way is important for the world of dermatology and skin care.

Ultimately, the Fitzpatrick scale classifies skin color by the way that different skin colors respond to sunlight, which is the most common form of ultraviolet (UV) radiation. The Fitzpatrick scale classifies skin color into six categories, from the lightest skin colors being Fitzpatrick type I to the darkest skin colors being Fitzpatrick type VI.

The lightest skin color category, Fitzpatrick type I, always burns and never tans in sunlight. This type of skin is pale and white, and people with this type of skin often have blue or green eyes as well as blond or red hair. People with Fitzpatrick type II skin also tend to be fair skinned, and they are categorized as burning easily and tanning poorly in sunlight. People with Fitzpatrick type III skin are typically able to tan but are still susceptible to burns and still have primarily white skin.

People with Fitzpatrick skin types IV, V, and VI are typically thought of as having skin of color because their primary skin color is more brown than white. People with Fitzpatrick type IV skin are able to tan easily with minimal burning, while people with Fitzpatrick type V skin rarely ever burn and tan darkly with mild sun exposure. Finally, people with the darkest skin color, Fitzpatrick type VI, have dark brown or Black skin and never burn but always tan darkly with sun exposure.

The distinction between the lighter skin types of Fitzpatrick I, II, and II as compared to darker skin types in Fitzpatrick IV, V, and VI is important when it comes to acne because of the way that acne is different in skin of color. The way that acne looks in those darker skin tones can be radically different than the way that it looks in lighter skin. For example, while acne in people with lighter skin types mostly looks like red bumps that are easy to see due to the lack of color in the surrounding skin, acne bumps in skin of color is more challenging to see because the skin is already darkly colored. Importantly, people with skin of color who have acne are more likely to have more active acne that requires more treatment and is more extensive or severe.

Besides these basic differences in how acne presents in lighter skin as compared to darker skin, one of the most profound differences in acne in different skin types is the impact that acne leaves behind after it heals. In lighter skin tones, when acne is treated early and appropriately, there is usually minimal change left in the skin once the acne bumps resolve.

However, in darker skin, acne can leave behind discoloration in the skin, which can be a huge source of distress for people with skin of color.

This phenomenon is called *postinflammatory hyperpigmentation*, which is a term that means that the inflammation from conditions like acne causes the skin to become more pigmented, or darkly colored, than the surrounding areas of unaffected skin. This causes the discoloration effect that is seen in people with skin of color who suffer from acne. The reason that this happens is because melanocytes, which are the cells in the skin responsible for producing the pigment that colors human skin, are very sensitive to inflammation and extreme changes in temperature. When inflammation occurs, the pigment production and even location of melanocytes in the skin is altered, causing the skin to change tone and become darker.

Additionally, people with skin of color are more prone to the development of keloids, which can be a big problem. While scars commonly occur following severe acne in any skin color, keloids are scars that grow in size and become larger than the original acne damage that caused the scarring. This can be very disfiguring and cause significant distress, especially when it occurs on the face or other sensitive body areas. Between the vulnerability of skin of color to postinflammatory hyperpigmentation and keloid formation, acne can have a much more severe impact on people with skin of color as compared to those with lighter skin types.

Unfortunately, there are also cultural differences in the experience of acne for people with skin of color. One study showed that Black patients were less likely to receive oral acne medications as compared to Caucasian patients, and that Black patients were also less frequently prescribed antibiotics, even when appropriate for managing their acne. This is just one troubling example among many that illustrates the challenges that people with skin of color face when seeking care for medical conditions such as acne. These differences in the quality of health care that people of color receive have also been seen in a variety of serious medical conditions, such as heart attacks, strokes, diabetes, and even pregnancy and childbirth.

10. What is the difference between acne and rosacea?

While acne is a very common and usually instantly recognizable skin condition, there are a number of other skin conditions that can look very similar to acne. The most common mimicker of acne is a skin condition called *rosacea*. In fact, this skin condition is so similar to acne that its full scientific name is *acne rosacea*. Although acne and rosacea can look very similar, they are different skin conditions, and there are subtle differences that can help in telling the two apart. This is important because the symptoms and treatment of rosacea are very different than in acne.

Rosacea is another one of the most common skin conditions that people experience, especially in the United States and other Western countries. In the United States, approximately 14 million people are estimated to suffer from rosacea. Worldwide, up to over 400 million people are thought to experience rosacea, making it one of the most common skin conditions in the world behind conditions such as acne and eczema.

The simplest form of rosacea is a tendency to blush or flush more easily than other people. The redness from this flushing or blushing typically affects the face, especially the nose and cheeks. However, as rosacea becomes more severe, the redness and flushing can affect other parts of the face and chest in striking ways. While there are multiple kinds of rosacea, the most common categories include rosacea with tiny visible blood vessels and rosacea with little bumps and breakouts. This latter form of rosacea can be very hard to tell apart from acne and is often confused for acne, which can be a big problem because the treatments for acne and rosacea are very different. Ultimately, the most reliable way to tell acne and rosacea apart is by looking for comedones, which is the scientific name for blackheads and whiteheads. While acne has blackheads and whiteheads, rosacea does not.

The redness seen in acne and rosacea can also be very different. In acne, the redness is caused by inflammation around acne bumps or pimples. Therefore, the redness is only in the pimple and surrounding skin. However, in rosacea, the redness is a result of skin flushing and blood vessels, so large patches of skin on the face can be red, even beyond the area immediately around the rosacea bumps. Additionally, the symptoms of rosacea are often suddenly triggered by things like exercise, eating spicy foods, sun exposure, and drinking alcohol. Therefore, rosacea redness usually appears quickly and then fades away within days, unlike acne, which has a steadier and more chronic course. Unfortunately, rosacea can also affect the eyes, causing eye redness, irritation, and burning, whereas acne does not affect the eyes.

Another important difference between acne and rosacea is the demographics of the people who it affects. Acne affects people of all races, ethnicities, and skin types, while rosacea is more common among people with fairer skin types. These are typically people with Fitzpatrick skin types I, II, and III. In addition, while acne typically begins during adolescence and can continue into early adulthood, rosacea more commonly begins at approximately age thirty in most people. While rosacea typically affects people at an older age than acne, the incidence of older adults experiencing acne for the first time has been increasing in recent decades.

One of the most important reasons for correctly identifying acne and rosacea is because the treatments for these two common skin conditions are quite different. In fact, many people are misdiagnosed and incorrectly treated because of the confusion between acne and rosacea, which delays their skin recovery.

For acne, the most common treatments involve skin hygiene and the use of medications that exfoliate the skin, regulate the turnover of skin, and target the overgrowth of bacteria. When these medications are not effective, an oral medication known as isotretinoin, or brand name Accutane, can be given with usually significant improvement over the course of weeks and months.

For rosacea, the most common treatments include topical medications that reduce redness and flushing by causing the blood vessels in the skin to constrict, or tighten. These medications are typically effective much more rapidly than acne medications but are temporary in their effect and require regular reapplication. In addition, other medications, such as metronidazole, are sometimes used to help treat rosacea bumps. Interestingly, oral antibiotics and sometimes even isotretinoin can be given to help with rosacea that is not responding well to common treatments. However, this is usually a second- or third-line option.

11. What other conditions can mimic acne?

Besides rosacea, there are a few other skin conditions that can look like acne and be challenging to tell apart. Some of these mimickers look like acne because of the areas of the skin that they affect, especially areas such as the face, while other mimickers share similar features with acne, including redness and bumps on the skin. Although these conditions may look very similar to acne, they are different in small or large ways, and it is possible to tell them apart based on their features and other characteristics.

Seborrheic dermatitis is another extremely common skin condition that can sometimes look similar to acne, especially because it mainly affects the areas of the skin that have lots of oil-producing glands, the same areas that acne affects. Seborrheic dermatitis is a skin condition that causes redness, itchiness, and greasy flaking of the skin in areas such as the scalp, face, and chest. It is thought to be caused by multiple factors, but an immune response to yeast that live on the skin is involved. Common dandruff is thought to be a mild form of seborrheic dermatitis, while the severe form can be very inflamed and uncomfortable for people. Although seborrheic dermatitis may look like acne because of its redness and location, the flaking skin in the affected area is a big clue that it is not acne. Additionally, treatment with antifungal creams and washes typically significantly improves the condition, which is a response that is not seen in people who have acne that try topical antifungal treatments.

In addition to seborrheic dermatitis, keratosis pilaris is another skin condition that can occasionally look similar to mild acne. Keratosis pilaris is a genetic condition that is extremely common, affecting at least half of adolescents and at least a third of adults. In keratosis pilaris, the skin follicles stick out more than usual, causing the skin to appear bumpy. This is sometimes referred to as looking like "chicken skin." Occasionally, the bumps of keratosis pilaris can become irritated and red, causing it look similar to acne, especially when it occurs on the face. However, unlike acne, keratosis pilaris usually looks uniform and regular in appearance because the majority of the follicles are affected. This is different than acne, where the red bumps often have different sizes and shapes because they develop at different times.

Folliculitis is another skin condition that can affect multiple hair follicles in an area of the skin, causing the skin to mimic the appearance of irritated acne. In folliculitis, there is a bacterial infection of multiple hair follicles that causes the appearance of red bumps, which can be itchy and uncomfortable. Sometimes, however, folliculitis can affect just one follicle, causing it to become a large red bump on its own. Folliculitis is commonly seen after shaving the legs or arms with a dirty razor or sitting in a hot tub that has not been appropriately cleaned. There are other forms of folliculitis that can be caused by viruses, fungi, and even mites, and these typically cause similar symptoms of itch, redness, and bumps on the skin. Ultimately, folliculitis will resolve fairly quickly in most people with the use of topical antibiotic creams placed on the skin over a period of days, unlike acne, which can take weeks to months to improve and requires multiple different types of medications and exfoliating creams.

Sebaceous hyperplasia is another skin condition that can occasionally look like acne. In sebaceous hyperplasia, the sebaceous glands—the oil-producing glands of the skin—become abnormally enlarged. *Hyperplasia* is one of the medical terms that is used to describe this enlargement beyond normal size. Therefore, in sebaceous hyperplasia, the oil glands can become enlarged and appear as bumps on the skin, mirroring mild acne. Of note, people do not usually experience sebaceous hyperplasia until they reach middle age, which is an important difference between sebaceous hyperplasia and acne, as acne more commonly affects adolescents and young adults.

Rarely, some skin cancers may mimic an acne pimple. For example, basal cell carcinoma, which is the most common skin cancer in the world, can grow into a nodule that sometimes looks similar to an acne bump. This can be a big problem in people who already have acne because some forms of basal cell carcinoma can be difficult to tell apart from the acne bumps that surround them. Some clues that what looks like an acne bump might be more concerning include continued growth despite treatment, easy bleeding on contact or shaving, and changes in appearance that do not match the other bumps on the skin. While basal cell carcinoma is a skin cancer that should be taken seriously and removed early, it does not typically spread to other areas of the body in the early stages and is usually completely cured with removal by a dermatologist.

The Causes of Acne

12. Why does acne happen?

There are many factors that interact to cause the whiteheads, blackheads, and other bumps on the skin that make up acne. Although much has been learned about these factors that contribute to causing acne, it is clear that acne is a complex condition and there is still a lot to learn regarding its causes.

The clearest pathway that leads to acne includes the blockage of hair follicles with natural skin oils from the skin's oil-producing glands and debris from dead skin cells. This blockage of the hair follicle is often thought to be due to an overproduction of natural skin oils because of factors like hormones or genetics. Hormones such as testosterone are powerful activators of the body's oil-producing sebaceous glands. When testosterone levels are high, such as during puberty or in medical conditions such as polycystic ovarian syndrome (PCOS), the sebaceous glands become activated and produce excess skin oils that can clog hair follicles. Additionally, some people are genetically prone to overproducing skin oils, and they can develop hair follicle blockage and acne during early adolescence or throughout adulthood.

The blockage of hair follicles can also occur due to a variety of other reasons. Touching or covering the skin, especially the skin of the face, can be a cause of hair follicle blockage in many people. Blocking the surface of the skin for extended periods of time, such as when wearing a mask for several hours or sleeping on a pillow facedown overnight, can prevent the natural skin oils from spreading normally and not allow the debris on the surface of the skin to be shed like usual, leading to blockage of hair follicles. There are also a variety of unhealthy skin-care routines and hygienic habits that can cause blockage of the hair follicles, including reusing dirty towels to clean the face and not changing pillowcases or masks that touch the skin frequently enough. The use of rough cleansers and the overapplication of lotions and moisturizers can also contribute to acne in people that are prone to it.

Whatever the particular reason that causes the hair follicle to become blocked might be, the ultimate result is that natural skin oils and skin debris fill and block the hair follicle, resulting in the whiteheads and blackheads that are characteristic of acne. Importantly, however, the presence of these whiteheads and blackheads does not lead to inflammation or redness in acne unless there is another factor that triggers inflammation, such as the overgrowth of bacteria that live on the skin.

The natural skin oils that block the hair follicle are the preferred food source of bacteria that live on the skin, especially a bacterium known as *Cutibacterium acnes*, or *C. acnes*. This bacterium is the primary bacteria involved in acne, and it consumes and digests the natural skin oils and produces by-products like free fatty acids. These by-products are strong triggers that cause inflammation in the skin, leading to the red bumps and irritation that are seen in more moderate to severe forms of acne. When inflammation is severe enough, the pimples and other red bumps of acne can become nodules or even cysts. Importantly, while the *C. acnes* species lives on the skin of almost all people, it typically does not cause any symptoms unless there is an excess of oil on the skin and blockage of hair follicles, as seen in acne. Also, it has been shown that there are some subtypes of the *C. acnes* species that are more likely to cause acne than other subtypes.

Beyond the pathway of hair follicle blockage and bacterial overgrowth, recent medical research has shown that genetics is responsible for a large portion of acne. In fact, up to 80% of the variation within the population for acne can be explained by genetics. There is not a single gene that is responsible, but a variety of genes involved in the inflammation process and regulation of skin have been found to contribute to an increased risk of acne in individuals. Therefore, if someone has parents or siblings with acne, his or her risk of developing acne is higher.

Acne is a complex condition that requires a variety of factors, including overproduction of skin oils, abnormal turnover of skin debris, blockage of hair follicles, overgrowth of bacteria, and the development of inflammation. There are a variety of subfactors that impact this pathway, including elevation of natural hormones in the body, such as testosterone; covering the skin for long periods of time; genetics; stress; diet; and a variety of medications. Therefore, acne is not caused by a single factor but rather the interaction of many different factors. Most likely, there are still a number of other factors that contribute to acne that are still waiting to be discovered by medical research.

13. How do hormones affect acne?

Hormones are one of the biggest causes of acne. Hormones are chemical messengers released by the body to control bodily functions such as growth, development, metabolism, and even mood. The body is able to adjust and adapt to different situations based on the levels of these hormones. For example, large shifts in hormone levels are responsible for signaling the beginning of puberty and the bodily changes that come with adolescence.

While there are a countless number of different chemicals that function as hormones in the human body, one of the most important categories responsible for contributing to acne is the androgen family. The androgens are a group of hormones that include testosterone, dehydroepiandrosterone (DHEA), and dihydrotestosterone (DHT), among many others, and they are responsible for regulating the development and maintenance of male characteristics during and following puberty. These male characteristics include an increase in the amount of muscle in the body, increased height growth, the development of body hair, and even changes in the brain and in brain functioning.

Important for its role in acne, the androgen hormones also play a large role in controlling the oil production of the body's sebaceous glands, which are responsible for producing the natural oils found on the skin. During puberty, the increased levels of testosterone and other androgens in the blood activate the sebaceous glands to produce significant amounts of oil. The oil is then emptied into the hair follicle so that it can rise to the top of the skin and provide a lubricating barrier.

However, since the levels of androgens during puberty can be very high and irregular, this process can lead to making too much skin oil, which can lead to clogging the hair follicle. Once the hair follicles are clogged, the blackheads and whiteheads of acne can be seen, and without treatment, pimples can form and acne can get worse. This is why acne is most frequently seen during puberty and adolescence and why it typically gets better as people end their teenage years and their body's androgen levels normalize.

Another subset of hormones that is involved in the development of acne includes estrogen and progesterone. While androgens are the hormones most responsible for male characteristics, estrogens play an important role in the development of female characteristics. These estrogens also oppose the effects of androgens on the body's sebaceous glands. While androgens activate the sebaceous glands, estrogens reduce the function and size of the sebaceous glands. Additionally, estrogen increases the production of sex hormone–binding globulin, which is a protein that can bind and hold on to testosterone to reduce the amount of testosterone available in the bloodstream. In this way, estrogen can reduce acne activity. On the other hand, the menstrual cycle also involves changes in progesterone levels in addition to estrogen, and it has been more recently discovered that progesterone has its own unique role in influencing the skin and contributing to flares of acne during the menstrual cycle.

In addition to androgens, estrogens, and progesterone, insulin and insulin-like growth factor are another group of important contributors to the development of acne. The cells that make up the sebaceous glands of the body are known as sebocytes, and these sebocytes have receptors for insulin on their surface. When insulin levels are increased, such as when lots of carbohydrates are eaten, the sebocytes respond by increasing the number of receptors on their surface for growth hormones. This makes the sebocytes and sebaceous glands more sensitive to growth factors in the body, which can cause the sebocytes to grow and be more active, resulting in more oil production and a higher chance of acne developing. This is how high-sugar foods that cause a lot of insulin release in the body can lead to the worsening of acne in people who are prone to the condition.

Glucocorticoids are another major group of hormones that play a role in controlling acne activity. Glucocorticoids, a family of steroids that are made by the body, are thought to increase acne exacerbations by increasing the genetic expression of inflammatory proteins such as toll-like receptor 2. This leads to an increase of other inflammatory proteins and the inflammation and immune problems that contribute to acne. Importantly, this pathway is thought to be responsible for the development of acne in athletes who take injectable steroid medications for competitive athletics or bodybuilding. In these people, acne can be severe and widespread, and it can continue despite treatment until the steroid injections are stopped.

Since acne has been found to be highly influenced by hormonal balances within the body, there has been increased research on the role of hormone-targeted medical therapies for the treatment of acne. For example, spironolactone, which blocks testosterone activity, is an oral medication that has become increasingly used in the treatment of acne with hormonal features, particularly in women with acne along the jawline who experience acne breakouts during their menstrual cycles. In people with this menstrual type of acne, oral contraceptives are another effective tool for regulating and normalizing hormone levels in the body to treat acne. As the influence of hormones in the development of acne has been increasingly better understood, the role of treatments targeted at these pathways has increased.

14. What medical conditions can cause acne?

In most people, acne happens without any serious underlying medical condition causing it. However, in a small number of people, acne can be the result of another disease that affects the skin or entire body. For these people, finding and treating the underlying disease is usually needed to help the acne get better.

Because hormones play such an important role in causing acne, medical conditions that impact hormone levels in the body are some of the most frequent causes of acne. Medical conditions that impact the body's hormones are called endocrine conditions because the endocrine system is the collection of organs in the body responsible for controlling hormone levels. Endocrine conditions that have been found to cause acne include polycystic ovarian syndrome (PCOS), Cushing syndrome, and androgen-secreting tumors, among other rarer diseases.

PCOS is one of the most common endocrine conditions that is associated with acne. In fact, PCOS is so common that it has been estimated to affect up to 10% of women in the world. PCOS is thought to be caused by a variety of factors, including genetics and environment, and the major risk factors for the condition are obesity, lack of exercise, and a family history of the disease. When women have PCOS, the hormone levels in their body are not regulated correctly, and they have high levels of a number of hormones, including testosterone. This can lead to the development of many small cysts in the ovaries as well as the development of acne on the face and other areas of the body. The high levels of testosterone are thought to cause overproduction of oil on the skin, leading to blockage of hair follicles in the same way that testosterone contributes to acne during puberty. Thankfully, women with PCOS often benefit from taking medications that block the action of testosterone and other androgen hormones, such as spironolactone and oral contraceptives. Additionally, some women experience resolution or significant improvement of their PCOS with weight loss or increased exercise.

Another endocrine disorder that can cause acne is known as Cushing syndrome. In this condition, the body generates too much of a hormone called cortisol. Cortisol is a steroid that can trigger the development of acne throughout the face and body, especially on the trunk. The acne caused by cortisol is difficult to treat, and people who suffer from Cushing's syndrome can experience other problems, such as obesity, fatigue, high blood pressure, and high blood sugar, as a result of chronic high levels of steroid in their blood. Importantly, Cushing's syndrome can also develop in people who take medical steroids for the management of other medical conditions over a long period of time.

Acne can also be caused by androgen-secreting tumors. In these tumors, there is an overgrowth of cells that produce androgens such as testosterone. This leads to overproduction of androgens and a change in the hormonal balance of the body. The most common androgen-secreting tumors involve organs such as the ovaries or testicles or parts of the adrenal glands, which are on top of the kidneys. While androgen-secreting tumors are relatively rare, they are sometimes responsible for the presence of acne in young children who would otherwise not have high androgen levels in their blood until they reached puberty. In these children, the presence of the androgen-secreting tumor causes early signs of puberty as young as four to six years old. When these symptoms are present at an abnormally early age, further investigation is often done with imaging tools such as CT scans or ultrasounds to search for the presence of androgen-secreting tumors.

In addition to endocrine conditions, there are a number of other medical conditions that affect the whole body and can appear with acne. Apert syndrome is a genetic condition that primarily causes the bones of the body to develop abnormally. However, in addition to the abnormal bone development, it can also cause acne to appear.

SAPHO syndrome—also known as synovitis-acne-pustulosis-hyperostosis-osteitis syndrome—can appear with acne, but it is not clear why. PAPA syndrome—which stands for pyogenic arthritis, pyoderma gangrenosum, and acne syndrome—involves mutations in the genes responsible for inflammation in the body and can result in abnormal inflammation in the joints and skin as well as acne, among a number of other body issues.

There are also a variety of medications and supplements that can contribute to the development of acne. When acne is caused by medications, it is sometimes labeled as *acne medicamentosa*. Some of the medications that most commonly cause acne include testosterone, progesterone, steroids, lithium, phenytoin, isoniazid, and halogens as well as vitamins B2, B6, and B12. When acne occurs due to medications, the medications should ideally be stopped with the supervision of a physician. Once the responsible medication is stopped, the acne will typically resolve on its own within weeks to months. However, sometimes an important medication that cannot be safely stopped is responsible for the acne, and in these situations, the medical acne can be treated with additional medications without discontinuing the responsible medication.

15. Can stress affect acne?

Many people who suffer from acne are aware that they experience flares of their acne during times of increased stress, whether it be from school, work, or their personal lives. This is because stress can contribute to causing acne. In fact, stress plays a significant role in influencing most of the functions of the body.

Recent research has shown that stress, especially when it is over a long period of time, can impact almost every organ of the body, including the musculoskeletal system and nerves, the heart, the endocrine system, the digestive system, and even the skin. Stress can cause the muscles of the body to tense and become uncomfortable or painful. It can strain the function of the heart and increase inflammation, which damages blood vessels and leads to vascular disease, leading to heart attack and stroke. Importantly, stress can change the balance of hormone levels in the body, which causes a variety of effects and is thought to be responsible for how stress contributes to acne flare-ups.

There are a number of medical research studies that have shown that stress causes acne to become worse or flare. One such study examined a group of university students and compared the severity of their acne during periods of low and high stress. This study found that students had worse acne during periods of higher stress, such as during their university exam weeks. Another study examining over 1,000 high school students found a similar association between acne worsening and periods of increased stress.

While the exact way that stress causes acne to flare is not yet known, there are a couple of different mechanisms that have been suspected to be responsible. One potential cause is an increase in the levels of androgens in the body as a result of stress. These androgens are then able to increase the size of sebaceous glands in the body and increase the amount of oils that they produce, leading to worsening of acne. Another potential pathway in which stress might make acne worse involves hormones such as glucocorticoids, which are steroids that similarly cause sebaceous glands to increase their oil production, which can lead to acne.

In addition, it is thought that high levels of stress can cause the release of proteins in the body that increase inflammation and lead to inflammation-related damage. This increased level of inflammation can damage blood vessels and lead to vascular disease, but it can also cause irritation and inflammation in the skin. This might be a particularly important pathway for people who already have acne who notice that their acne becomes redder and more inflamed during periods of high stress. Unfortunately, this inflammation can also lead to the release of chemicals such as substance P, which can activate sebaceous glands to produce more natural skin oils, which, in turn, worsen acne.

Interestingly, the power of stress to impact the function of skin is highlighted by the observation during research studies that psychological stress can slow the healing of skin wounds by up to 40%. Therefore, while the exact way that stress influences the skin and worsens acne is not yet known, it is clear that there is a strong relationship between stress and acne.

16. How does weight gain affect acne?

The relationship between weight and acne is a topic that has been very controversial over the past decade. In fact, multiple research studies have been carried out, and these studies have found different and opposite results. Despite this, weight and acne have been found to be related to each other in a number of ways.

Weight can be measured through a couple of different methods, but one of the most common ways to measure and understand weight is through the body mass index (BMI), which is a number that is calculated by using an individual's weight and height. This allows a person's weight to be understood in comparison with his or her height, since taller individuals are often heavier than shorter individuals. The concept of BMI is particularly important to understand because most of the research studies that have explored the relationship between acne and weight have used BMI rather than directly using weight.

The current recommendations from the CDC state that a BMI between 18.5 and 24.9 indicates a healthy weight. BMI numbers below this range indicate that a person is underweight, and BMI numbers above this range indicate that a person is overweight or obese. Importantly, this is still an imperfect way of categorizing body weight because BMI does not account for differences between muscle and fat, and muscle is denser than fat, which can result in lean athletes or large bodybuilders being classified as overweight or obese because they have a lot of muscle mass. Although BMI is imperfect, it can still be a useful tool for the medical field and scientific research.

There have been several large research studies that have tried to examine whether the rate of acne increases as BMI increases or whether having a larger relative body weight is protective against acne. While some research studies found that weight or BMI did not impact the rate of acne, one of the largest studies that has been done found that the rate of acne went down as BMI increased. This means that being overweight or obese was found to be associated with a decreased rate of acne. While this is a controversial finding, the study that showed this was one of the most extensive studies ever done on the topic. It included over 600,000 youth, giving it significant power. It found that up to 20% of underweight youth experienced acne, while only up to 14% of severely obese youth reported having acne.

While the findings of this large study were surprising given the long-standing belief that obesity makes acne worse rather than protects against it, there are a couple of caveats to be aware of. Importantly, a lot of foods, such as refined items, sugary foods, sugar-sweetened beverages, and dairy-heavy foods, are associated with contributing to both acne and weight gain. So, while someone who may be overweight or obese might have a lower risk of developing acne than someone who is underweight, the quality of the food that they eat and the food choices that they are able to make can still increase their risk of developing acne.

In addition, while the rate of acne might decrease as weight increases, the severity of acne has been clearly shown to be much worse in people who are obese. This is particularly a problem in those who have very high BMIs and develop very severe acne with nodules, cysts, and extensive involvement of their face, body, and limbs. Also, people who have higher BMIs have been shown to experience the inflammatory form of acne more commonly than those with lower BMIs. Therefore, the relationship between weight and acne is far from simple.

Interestingly, it is not only weight that plays a role in the development of acne but also the rate of weight change. In people who lose weight rapidly, there can be large shifts in hormone levels in the body. This change in hormone balance can contribute to the sudden appearance of acne and even hair loss in some people.

In addition, there are a number of medical conditions that connect weight and acne. For example, polycystic ovarian syndrome (PCOS) is strongly associated with being overweight and often manifests with acne. PCOS is a very common medical condition affecting women and is thought to be caused by an imbalance of hormones in the body. Therefore, in some select people, having a higher weight can be associated with contributing to acne.

17. Do alcohol and smoking influence acne?

It is commonly thought that alcohol and smoking contribute to acne and can significantly worsen the condition. Surprisingly, alcohol has never been shown to directly affect acne. However, smoking has been directly linked with causing and worsening acne in significant ways.

There have been a number of studies that examined the relationship between alcohol and acne, but there has never been an association between alcohol and acne that has been discovered. Importantly, however, in extreme situations where alcohol intake is excessive, it can cause damage to internal organs like the liver and change the balance of hormones and other chemicals in the body. Also, excessive alcohol intake can contribute to dehydration. These factors may potentially contribute to the development of acne and other skin conditions. For most people who have a low to moderate intake of alcohol, this is not a concern, and alcohol does not cause acne or contribute to the development of acne breakouts.

Smoking, on the other hand, has been strongly linked with the presence and severity of acne. In fact, smoking has been shown to negatively impact almost every single aspect of physical health, from the brain to the heart and to the skin.

The impact that smoking has on the skin is significant. Smoking causes the skin to age faster than normal, resulting in wrinkling and dryness. It causes wounds to heal more slowly throughout the body, and it increases the risk for skin infections to develop. Importantly, smoking also contributes to a higher risk for many different skin conditions, including acne, psoriasis, and even lupus.

Smoking and skin disease might be related in a variety of ways. Smoking causes toxic chemicals to enter the body, and smoking nicotine can cause a process called oxidative stress, which can directly damage the skin's blood vessels and collagen supply and lead to significant inflammation. Even smoking nicotine-free substances such as marijuana can contribute to the development of skin disease, as the act of smoking reduces oxygen levels in the blood and can lead to oxidative stress.

Research studies have shown that smoking in general increases the risk for developing acne. This increased risk of acne in people who smoke continues into late adulthood, with people between the ages of twenty-five and fifty being much more likely to develop acne if they smoke than if they do not smoke.

Importantly, smoking has also been found to be associated with an increased severity of acne when it does occur. For people who smoke, acne is more likely to involve a larger amount of skin area and feature more pimples. In fact, smoking can be a common trigger for acne breakouts in people who otherwise have milder forms of acne. Therefore, stopping smoking can be a very important part of the treatment of acne in people who struggle with nicotine addiction and other smoking behaviors.

The process of stopping smoking, known as smoking cessation, is very challenging, however. Nicotine and other substances can be extremely addictive to the brain, leading to dependence on frequent smoking. For people who develop an addiction to smoking nicotine, stopping can lead to withdrawal symptoms, significant discomfort, and even pain. This can make smoking cessation difficult for many people. However, there are a variety of tools that can help in making quitting nicotine easier, including nicotine replacement gums, nicotine patches, and even psychological counseling. In fact, one of the biggest factors that determines whether someone can successfully quit smoking is the number of times that they have attempted to quit smoking. The more times someone attempts to quit smoking, the more likely they are to eventually succeed, even if all the prior attempts resulted in failure.

Once an individual quits smoking, the negative effects described earlier can begin to disappear, and the severity of acne begins to improve. There are some long-term or lifelong effects that cannot be reversed, such as some of the early aging effects on the skin and the increased risk of multiple forms of cancer, but many of the negative impacts of smoking improve with time after smoking cessation, including the risk for worse acne.

18. How does diet affect acne?

The connection between diet and acne has become more obvious in the modern era. A variety of foods and diets have been linked to affecting acne in people who are prone to the condition. Although some foods have been debunked as causing acne, there is still a wide variety of foods that have shown to have an influence on making acne better or worse. Food and diet are not the only factors that cause acne, but they play a role in combination with many other factors.

The glycemic index is one of the major concepts that has been found to connect food and acne. The glycemic index is a measure of how quickly individual foods increase the level of sugar in the bloodstream. Foods high on the glycemic index cause rapid increases in blood sugar levels, while foods low on the glycemic index raise blood sugar levels slowly. Refined sugars, white bread, pasta, and white rice are examples of high glycemic index foods, while whole wheat breads and protein-rich foods typically have a lower glycemic index.

The glycemic index of foods is important because faster rises in blood sugar levels cause hormone levels in the body to change in significant ways. When a person eats high glycemic index foods, the level of sugar in their bloodstream rises rapidly, and this triggers significant increases in the levels of insulin, growth hormone, and other hormones in the body. These hormones can have a large influence on acne and result in worsening acne when they are increased by high glycemic index foods.

One study of several thousand Americans who were placed on a low-glycemic diet found that it reduced acne in a significant and clinically meaningful way. Almost nine out of ten people on the low-glycemic diet reported having less acne and required less acne medication for treating their acne. Other medical studies from Australia, Korea, and Turkey also found that a low-glycemic diet significantly lessened acne.

It is believed that low glycemic index foods reduce acne by reducing spikes in blood sugar levels. These spikes impact hormone levels and can lead to increased inflammation throughout the body. In addition, blood sugar spikes can also cause the oil production of the skin to abnormally increase, which is a risk factor for developing acne. Therefore, since low-glycemic foods do not cause as many blood sugar level spikes, inflammation and oil production may decrease to normal levels and contribute to the improvement of acne.

Another category of food associated with acne in the modern era is dairy, or products created from cow's milk. In one medical research study, women who drank two or more glasses of cow's milk per day were found to be almost 50% more likely to have acne than women who did not drink as much cow's milk. Other studies in the United States, Italy, and Malaysia have found similar results.

While the relationship behind how cow's milk might make acne worse is still rather unclear, there are a variety of potential causes that have been proposed. Some of these potential mechanisms include hormones from cow's milk leading to hormonal imbalance in the body, proteins from cow's milk leading to increased inflammation in the skin and other areas of the body, and proteins in cow's milk stimulating the increased production of natural hormones in the body. While each of these mechanisms are reasonable, none of them have been definitively shown to be responsible. Additionally, processed dairy in the form of cheeses and yogurts has not been shown to be associated with acne.

Chocolate is another category of food that has been suggested as an acne trigger, especially in popular culture. Interestingly, this association has not been clearly proven despite many research studies on the topic. One research study found that acne worsened in a group of young adult men after eating 100% cocoa powder capsules every day for two weeks. At the same time, however, other research studies have found no link between chocolate and acne. It is unclear how chocolate might be connected with worsening acne, but some proposed mechanisms include chocolate increasing the sensitivity of the immune system to the skin bacteria involved in acne. Therefore, while some people might want to limit their chocolate intake as part of treating their acne, it is not likely to play a large role in the process.

Another major concept connecting food and acne is food sensitivity. Food sensitivity is when an individual is sensitive to a certain category of food, such as tree nuts, mushrooms, or certain fruits or vegetables. When ingesting the food, the individual's immune system is activated, causing irritation, discomfort, and widespread inflammation. The widespread inflammation can then contribute to the development and flaring of acne on the skin.

Importantly, however, food sensitivities are different than allergies. In allergies, there is an immediate immune system response to certain foods that can cause hives across the skin, swelling of the lips and throat, and even death in severe cases. While allergies and food sensitivities are often caused by similar types of food, food insensitivities tend to be more long term and present with less immediate symptoms.

In people who suffer from food sensitivities, an elimination diet supervised by trained health-care and dietitian experts can be a powerful tool for identifying and removing trigger foods. In an elimination diet, the diet is significantly simplified so that most potential triggers are removed. Then, foods are slowly added back into the diet one by one until the food sensitivity symptoms return, allowing the most recently added food to be identified as a trigger for food sensitivity. It is important to do elimination diets under the supervision of a trained and certified health-care professional to ensure adequate nutrition and health while limiting the variety of foods that are eaten.

In addition to foods that can cause or worsen acne, there are a variety of foods and nutrients that might contribute to improving acne. The majority of these foods are thought to help control and improve acne by managing and controlling inflammation in the body. These foods and nutrients include omega-3 fatty acids, green tea, turmeric, and certain vitamins and minerals. Additionally, diets such as the paleo diet, which involves eating mostly lean meats and vegetables, and the Mediterranean diet, which involves primarily eating seafood, whole wheats, and fruits and vegetables, have been found to show a beneficial effect on acne.

However, it is important to understand that while diet changes can help in managing acne, they are not a replacement for medical therapy, which remains the most effective and important treatment for acne.

19. Can wearing makeup cause acne?

Makeup can definitely contribute to acne. In fact, acne that is caused by makeup is sometimes referred to by its own special medical term: *acne cosmetica*. Acne cosmetica, or acne caused by makeup, can happen to anyone, but it most frequently occurs in women. In acne cosmetica, the skin of the face usually develops lots of tiny bumps on the cheeks, chin, forehead, or other areas where makeup is typically placed. In people with acne breakouts around the lips, lipstick or lip balm can sometimes be the culprit.

Acne cosmetica can occur within a few days after using makeup, or it may take several months to develop after repeated applications of makeup. Therefore, it may be difficult to suspect makeup as the culprit causing the acne, especially in situations where the acne develops a long time after a certain makeup product has been used.

There are a variety of factors that can determine which makeup products cause acne and which ones do not. One of the most important factors responsible for makeup causing acne is the ingredient list used to develop the makeup. There are a variety of ingredients in makeup, especially foundation, that can contribute to worsening acne. Chemicals such as isopropyl myristate, sodium lauryl sulfate, myristyl myristate, and laureth-4 can irritate the skin or clog the skin pores, which can cause or worsen acne. Additionally, foundations made with alcohol can be drying to the skin, while those made with oils can clog pores.

In addition to avoiding common irritating and pore-clogging ingredients, it is important to understand and avoid personal sensitivities. Each individual's skin is different, and while a particular makeup product might not have common acne-causing ingredients, it can still cause acne if the user is sensitive to a specific ingredient in the makeup. Therefore, being attentive to which makeup products trigger acne is an important part of using makeup in a responsible and mindful way.

Even in situations where makeup products are appropriately chosen and do not have acne-causing ingredients, leaving makeup on the skin for long periods of time without removing it can still lead to acne breakouts and worsening of acne bumps. While some foundation makeups include ingredients that attempt to prevent acne from developing, leaving foundation on the skin for a long period of time can block the normal shedding of skin debris and cause a buildup of skin oils on the surface of the skin. Therefore, one of the most common reasons that makeup triggers acne is the long-term use of makeup, such as foundation, without daily cleansing of the skin and removal of the makeup, especially at night before sleeping.

Another common way that makeup can contribute to acne is through the tools that are used to apply makeup, like makeup brushes and applicators. These tools play a very important role in applying makeup to the skin; therefore, it is important to frequently clean and change them. When individuals reuse makeup brushes and applicators without appropriately cleaning them, it can cause skin debris, oils, and other pore-clogging materials to build up, which can worsen acne. This is especially problematic when sharing makeup and tools with other people.

While it is important to frequently clean makeup application tools, it is not a good idea to replace makeup application tools with the use of fingers and hands. Many people find it easiest to apply makeup with their fingertips, which can be a trigger for acne, since the hands are a skin location with many natural oils that can be transferred to the face and worsen acne.

20. Is acne caused by poor hygiene?

Poor hygiene can be a minor contributor to acne in some people who are prone to developing acne, but it does not cause acne on its own. This is an important point to understand because most people still hold on to the myth that acne is primarily caused by dirty skin or poor hygiene habits. In fact, one study found that over 90% of surveyed students believed that dirt and poor hygiene are responsible for acne. However, this could not be further from the truth. Poor hygiene can make acne worse, but the person has to have acne or be prone to acne in the first place for poor hygiene to play a role.

There have been multiple studies comparing people who wash their face once, twice, or four times a day to see whether frequency of cleaning the skin and hygiene habits impact acne. In these studies, there has not been any difference in the appearance of acne found between people. Therefore, it does not seem that hygiene plays a major role in the development of acne in most people. In fact, most dermatologists recommend against face washing more frequently than twice a day because it can be irritating to skin and even be a trigger for an acne breakout itself.

However, the origin of the myth that poor hygiene causes acne can be easily imagined. Since acne is a skin condition caused by excess skin oil production, abnormal shedding of dead skin cells, and the overgrowth of normal skin bacteria, it makes sense that poor hygiene can impact acne by worsening all of those factors. However, this has not been shown to be the case for a number of reasons. In fact, most of the processes responsible for acne are outside of the control of people who suffer from acne. For example, no matter how frequently they wash their skin, people with acne will still experience abnormal skin oil production because these problems begin from the inside of the skin rather than the surface of the skin. Additionally, the role of hormones and genetics largely outweighs the influence of smaller factors such as hygiene, diet, and other contributors.

While hygiene only plays a small role in the development of most cases of acne, there are indeed some situations in which hygiene can actually play a more meaningful role in causing or worsening acne. One of the most common of these situations is exercise and sweat. Wearing tight-fitting clothing that does not let sweat leave the skin during exercise can contribute to making acne worse. It is also usually recommended to shower immediately after exercise so that sweat, dirt, and excess oils on the skin are cleaned away and are not able to clog skin pores or worsen acne. However, this advice has been controversial since one study showed that there was no difference in the acne of people who showered immediately after exercise and those who delayed showering until several hours after exercise. In addition, removing makeup prior to exercise is important because it prevents skin pores from becoming clogged, which can be a risk factor for worsening acne.

For those who engage in sports and group exercise, another important hygiene habit that can influence acne is avoiding sharing protective equipment like helmets and shoulder pads when possible. Shared exercise equipment is often preworn and dirty, and it can contain dirt and oils that worsen acne when worn.

While it is important to maintain clean hygiene for a variety of reasons, the link between hygiene and acne is minimal in most situations.

However, many people can take the connection to an extreme by attempting to "clean" their way out of having acne. This typically involves heavy skin scrubbing with harsh soaps and cleansers, overly frequent bathing with hot water, and other excessive cleaning behaviors. Ironically, these hygiene habits may actually be harmful to the skin and lead to irritation and dryness, which can lead to acne flares in some situations. Therefore, it is important to keep hygiene habits in moderation without taking them to an extreme in either direction. Additionally, for those who do have acne, it is important to get care for their skin through a primary care doctor or a dermatologist rather than trying to treat their acne just by changing their hygiene habits.

21. Is there a genetic component to acne?

Genetics play a large role in many medical conditions, including acne. In fact, a person's genetic background has been found to be one of the biggest risk factors in determining his or her risk of developing acne.

All life on earth is influenced by genes; they form the foundation of genetics. Genes are the microscopic pieces of DNA and RNA that code all the instructions needed for the body to build and maintain human life. These genes often code for the construction of proteins and other molecules that form the bodies of all organisms, from bacteria, to animals, to human beings. These genes are also crucial for the passing of traits and attributes from one generation to another, including features like eye color, skin tone, hair color, and even a number of medical conditions.

While some traits, like having a widow's peak or freckles, are controlled by a single gene, most traits are controlled by a lot of different genes that interact with each other. In the case of acne, there is a large number of genes that has been found to contribute to the risk of developing acne. These genes produce proteins that function in different ways to maintain the health of the skin, and when these genes vary from normal, they can increase the risk of developing acne.

Most of the genes that have been found to be related to acne are genes that code for proteins involved in inflammation in the body. These genes include those that code for the proteins known as tumor necrosis factor (TNF), interleukin (IL), and toll-like receptor 4 (TLR4). These different proteins have many varying functions in the body, but their most important roles involve controlling and influencing the body's immune system response. While every human being has genes that code for these proteins, each individual's genetic code is slightly different, and this can influence the function of their proteins. In some of these individuals, minor differences in their proteins can increase their risk of developing acne. Importantly, since these proteins are coded by genes, and genes can be passed on from parents to their children, the risk for acne is something that can be passed down through families.

Interestingly, a variety of medical research has supported the view that acne is largely genetic in nature. One way to tell whether a medical condition can be inherited through genes is to compare how frequently identical twins share the condition and how frequently nonidentical twins share the condition. Because identical twins share the same exact genetic code and nonidentical twins share only portions of the same genetic code, medical conditions that are genetic in nature will be more commonly shared by identical twins than by nonidentical twins.

In acne, the results of these studies among twins found that 50%–90% of acne was due to genetics in affected people. Supporting this result was the finding that nearly half of twins with acne had at least one sibling with acne, while only about one in ten twins without acne had a sibling with acne. In addition, certain populations of people are more likely to develop acne; specifically, a study of teenage Americans of European origin found that this group of people have a risk of developing acne that is almost two and a half times higher than the general population. This increased rate of acne is thought to be due to genetic differences between that population and the general population.

Although there has been a lot of evidence discovered through modern medical research supporting the view that acne is greatly influenced by genetics, it is important to understand that genetics are not the only determining factor in people with acne. Genetic differences in people with acne simply create a higher likelihood of developing acne than the general population. There are still a variety of important factors that determine whether people who are genetically vulnerable to acne will develop the condition. These factors include hormone levels, especially during puberty, as well as stress, diet, and many others. Therefore, while genetics plays an important role in determining the risk for acne, it is far from being the only factor responsible.

22. How does pregnancy influence acne?

Hormones are one of the biggest and most influential factors that impact acne. This is because a lot of the cells and structures involved in acne, including the oil-producing glands and the hair follicles, are strongly controlled and influenced by hormone signals in the body. It is no wonder then that pregnancy, with all of the huge hormonal changes that accompany it, can influence acne in a significant way.

Even prior to pregnancy, the menstrual cycle involves an ever-changing cycle of hormone levels in the female body. Due to these constant changes in hormone levels, many women experience acne linked with their menstrual cycle. It is thought that menstrual acne is specifically caused by the sudden drop of estrogen and progesterone levels that happens immediately before the beginning of the menstrual cycle or period. This sudden drop causes the oil production of the skin to increase, leading to acne. In addition, this sharp change in hormone levels can also lead to inflammation that can worsen acne.

However, once pregnancy occurs, the hormone changes in the body can increase by even more than the changes seen in the menstrual cycle. Increased levels of estrogen, progesterone, and many other hormones can influence the skin and other organs in profound ways. In fact, about half of women develop some degree of acne during pregnancy due to these large hormone changes.

While the acne of pregnancy can follow different cycles, the most common timeline is that pregnant women experience a flare of acne during the first trimester. This is because the levels of progesterone surge to one of their highest levels at that time, primarily because those high levels of progesterone are needed to signal the uterus to create an accommodating environment for the fetus. Typically, the body's hormone levels tend to stabilize throughout the second and third trimesters, allowing acne to slowly improve, but this varies from woman to woman. Some women continue to experience acne flares throughout their pregnancy.

Unfortunately, the acne that occurs in pregnancy can also be different than classic acne. While classic acne is similarly influenced by hormones, it is also influenced by other factors, such as diet and stress. However, pregnancy acne is not as influenced by these factors; therefore, lifestyle changes are not as effective in improving the acne of pregnancy. In addition, the most commonly used medications that help with severe acne in most people are not safe to use in pregnancy, specifically retinoid-based medications such as isotretinoin, also known as Accutane. Therefore, the acne of pregnancy can be much harder to effectively treat compared to typical acne.

When the baby is born and the body's state of pregnancy is completed, the hormone changes associated with childbearing are far from over, especially in women who choose to breastfeed. In fact, hormone levels in the weeks to months following childbirth can still be different than normal. This is why the period after childbirth is sometimes referred to as the "fourth trimester"—because the body is still adapting to a different level of hormone function. In women who breastfeed, the act of nursing can be a powerful trigger of hormones that can sometimes contribute to the development of acne flares. In addition, medications and other chemicals can be transferred through the breastmilk from mother to baby. Therefore, some of the stronger acne medications still cannot be used by nursing mothers, even though their pregnancy is otherwise over.

Most of the medications that are not safe to use during pregnancy belong to a class of medications called retinoids. These medications are highly effective at controlling acne and improving the condition of the skin, but they have been associated with an increased risk of certain birth defects. Therefore, retinoids cannot be used during pregnancy. In fact, people who take an oral form of retinoid medication are often required to use multiple forms of birth control to make sure that they do not become pregnant while they are on the medication. In addition, acne medications that lower hormone levels, such as the medication known as spironolactone, are also unsafe to use during pregnancy because hormone levels are very important for ensuring a healthy and successful pregnancy and altering levels of hormones can pose an unnecessary risk to the developing baby.

However, despite these limitations in acne treatments for pregnant and nursing women, there are still many acne medications that are entirely safe to use during pregnancy. There are many topical medications that are applied directly to the skin in the forms of creams, washes, and gels that can help improve acne in pregnant women. A variety of these medications, such as benzoyl peroxide and salicylic acid, help to exfoliate the skin and improve acne bumps, and they are entirely safe to use in pregnancy. In addition, topical antibiotics that are applied to the skin can be immensely helpful, especially in pregnant women who have red and irritated acne bumps on their face and body. Interestingly, laser and ultraviolet (UV) light treatments can also be an effective treatment during pregnancy when other medications are not desired. However, it is always important for pregnant women to consult with a doctor before making treatment decisions for their acne.

23. What medications can cause or worsen acne?

Although acne is a skin condition that benefits from treatment with a variety of medications, there are also a lot of medications that can contribute to acne or make the condition worse. Acne due to medications is a common enough problem that it has its own name, *acne medicamentosa*, which is a medical term derived from Latin.

A great number of medications can cause acne medicamentosa, and there are several different pathways by which these medications contribute to worsening acne. One of the most common medication groups that causes acne is steroids. These steroids include oral corticosteroids, which are medications used to treat a variety of diseases and conditions, such as inflammation, organ failure, and asthma, and injectable anabolic steroids, which are used to stimulate the growth of muscle mass in the body. These steroids can cause significant shifts in the hormonal balance of the body, and they can directly, as well as indirectly, trigger increased oil gland activity in the skin, leading to acne. Additionally, steroids can change the activity and behavior of bacteria on the surface of the skin, leading to inflammation and skin infections.

The acne caused by steroids may look different than classic acne. Although classic acne most commonly affects the face in most people and features multiple bumps of different shapes, steroid-caused acne usually involves dome-shaped bumps that are identical in shape and size. Additionally, the bumps of steroid-induced acne typically affect the chest in a significant way, which is less commonly seen in typical acne.

Although the acne seen in people who regularly use steroid medications can be severe, it usually resolves once the steroid medications are stopped. When this is not possible, such as in situations where people require steroids to treat serious medical conditions, treatment of the acne with acne medications can be beneficial, but this is sometimes less effective than in classic acne.

In addition to steroid-induced acne, other hormonal medications can play a significant role in worsening acne. These hormonal medications include a variety of birth control medications, such as IUDs and oral contraceptives. The impact that these medications have on the menstrual cycle and the body's hormonal balance can sometimes help in improving hormonal acne, but they can also sometimes worsen regular acne. Thankfully, most of the newer hormonal medications used for birth control have been developed to be more targeted and are less likely to cause acne to develop or worsen. However, when women who take birth control experience acne, finding a new method of birth control that works for them is an important part of treating their acne.

There are also various medications used to treat neurologic medical conditions that can contribute to worsening acne. These medications are used to treat conditions such as seizures, depression, anxiety, and bipolar disorder. Lithium, carbamazepine, and sodium valproate are among the most commonly used neurologic medications that can induce acne in people who are prone to the condition. Lithium, for example, is thought to cause neutrophils—important immune system cells in the body—to move from the bloodstream into the skin, where they can cause inflammation and worsen acne. In many situations, this form of acne can become severe and be difficult to treat with the usual acne medications. However, stopping the responsible medication can be very challenging, especially when it is important for the treatment of serious conditions like seizure disorder or bipolar disorder.

In addition to the common medications that can cause acne, there are other substances that can worsen acne in people who have been exposed to them. Halogens are one common example of this. Halogens are substances composed of the chemicals fluoride, chloride, or bromide. People most commonly become exposed to halogens through work exposure and exposure through the environment. Those who work in fields related to industrial waste management, textiles, water management, the military, and chemical manufacturing are the most likely to be exposed to halogens on a regular basis. Unfortunately, exposure to halogens can lead to a severe form of acne that is referred to as *chloracne*. This form of acne can be more severe than regular acne and features significant redness and cysts that affect large areas of the body, including the chest, arms, and face. Unfortunately, halogens can remain in the body for a long period of time, and chloracne can take years to slowly improve. In fact, while chloracne usually improves over the course of two to three years, some people still experience the effects of halogen exposure for over fifteen years. In many patients, especially those with cysts and inflammation from chloracne, there can be significant scarring that never fully recovers.

Interestingly, a variety of supplements, vitamins, and minerals can also contribute to the development of acne. Rarely, B vitamins, including vitamin B6 and vitamin B12, have been found to increase the presence of acne in some people. When people take vitamin B6 or vitamin B12 supplements, the level of the vitamin in the skin has been observed to increase. This causes bacteria on the skin to release more porphyrins, which are a group of chemicals that can increase inflammation and worsen acne. In addition, some supplements may contain contaminants that can contribute to acne, especially because supplements in the United States are not held to the same purity standards as prescription medications.

24. What are some red flags that indicate a more serious form of acne?

The overwhelming majority of cases of acne are simple, uncomplicated acne that benefits from treatment with acne medications. However, on rare occasions, acne can sometimes be connected to a broader, more serious medical condition. In these situations, acne can be one of the first and most visible signs of serious illness. In addition, there are a few different acne syndromes that are associated with serious illnesses and have a number of characteristic symptoms.

There are some red flags that may indicate the presence of a more serious form of acne. While typical acne has a wide range of severity, from mild pimples on the skin to severe red bumps and cysts, the more serious forms of acne are usually striking in their appearance. Acne that is associated with syndromes such as PAPA syndrome (an acronym for pyogenic arthritis, pyoderma gangrenosum, and acne syndrome) or SAPHO syndrome (an acronym for synovitis-acne-pustulosis-hyperostosis-osteitis syndrome) can involve widespread areas of skin, including the face, chest, and back. In these areas, the acne can be extremely cystic, red, and painful. In fact, the acne can be so severe in these serious forms that it can be associated with fever, muscle aches, and joint pain. Acne in these serious conditions can be permanently disfiguring and cause a lot of physical and emotional anguish.

In addition to the severe appearance of the acne in these serious syndromes, there are often other accompanying symptoms that can hint to the presence of an underlying condition. For example, in SAPHO syndrome, the presence of severe acne is accompanied by joint inflammation, pustules throughout the body, and bone abnormalities. In PAPA syndrome, joint pain and the presence of lesions that look like deep ulcers are seen alongside the severe acne. When acne is accompanied by these specific conditions, it can indicate the presence of a more serious underlying syndrome.

Another major red flag is a lack of a response to treatment. Most forms of acne are able to be effectively treated with topical and oral acne medications. However, when acne does not respond to the normal acne medications, it can indicate either a more severe form of the disease or the presence of acne related to a broader medical condition. For example, in acne related to chronic steroid use, the acne often does not improve despite treatment with topical and oral medications. It is only after the underlying steroid use is addressed that the acne slowly improves and resolves. Additionally, in serious conditions such as chloracne, which is caused by halogens, acne can progressively worsen until the exposure to halogen substances is stopped—only then does the acne slowly improve over a long period of time.

While there are a variety of medical professionals that can diagnose and treat simple acne, there are a number of red flags that indicate that a dermatologist should be involved in the treatment. These red flags include the presence of severe acne with cysts, acne that has not responded to medications after three to six months, and acne that has scarring or that has caused significant emotional or psychological distress. It is important for dermatologists to be involved in the care of people with acne with these red flags because late treatment by dermatologists in these cases can result in permanent skin scarring and lifelong changes to the skin. By involving a dermatologist in the early treatment of acne with these signs, scarring can be avoided, and the acne can be treated effectively and efficiently.

The presence of psychological and emotional distress is another important red flag for anyone with acne to understand and look out for. Because acne often affects visible areas of the skin, such as the face, even mild forms of acne can cause distress and self-esteem issues. This is worsened by the fact that acne often occurs during adolescence, when individuals are sensitive to changes in their appearance and others' perceptions of them. In serious situations, this psychological and emotional suffering can extend to the point of depression, anxiety, and even suicidal thoughts. The presence of these feelings and thoughts is a red flag that someone with acne should seek medical attention and treatment, both because these feelings are not healthy and also because acne is usually treatable. Although acne is primarily a condition that affects the skin, the psychological impact of acne is increasingly being appreciated as an important part of the disease.

Living with Acne

25. How does acne impact self-image?

There are few medical conditions that can impact self-image as easily as acne. This is because acne usually happens on the most visible parts of the human body, such as the skin of the face. Also, acne typically happens during some of the most sensitive times of human development, such as adolescence and early adulthood, which are also the times most crucial to the growth of self-image. Therefore, acne has a profound ability to impact self-image in a variety of ways.

An individual's self-image includes the way that an individual views himself or herself as well as the way he or she believes others view him or her. While self-image includes many different facets, including personality and intelligence, physical appearance is a usually a major component of self-image. A person's self-image can influence the way that he or she feels, thinks, and views himself or herself and his or her role in the world. Therefore, self-image is a tremendously important part of human identity and purpose.

Due to the importance of self-image and the deep impact that acne can have on it, a lot of medical research has been done over the past decade or so to understand the ways that acne influences self-image. These research studies have discovered a number of fascinating findings. For example, nearly 30% to 50% of adolescents with acne report some form of psychological impact from having acne. The presence of acne in adolescents has also been associated with an increased rate of depression and anxiety. In one study, nearly a third of adolescents with acne suffered from depression or anxiety, while less than a tenth of adolescents without acne reported being depressed or anxious. Also, in those that suffer from acne, the rate of suicidal thoughts can be as high as 6%–7%, which is greatly disturbing. It has been shown that the psychological impact of acne is often worse the more severe the acne is.

Nearly all adolescents who suffer from acne report that they have felt embarrassed or self-conscious because of their acne. Almost two-thirds of adolescents with acne felt bothered by the appearance of their skin when they had acne. Importantly, those who had acne on the face were more likely to feel this way than those who had acne on other parts of the body, reinforcing the fact that the visibility of the skin of the face is one of the biggest reasons why acne can be so distressing.

Those with acne have also been found to have lower self-attitude, more feelings of uselessness, fewer feelings of pride, lower self-worth, and lower body satisfaction than those without acne. While acne has been shown to influence the self-image of women more negatively than men, it is important to understand that acne can negatively affect both men and women in profound ways.

Sadly, the impact that acne has on self-image can also influence the ways that people interact with those around them. Almost two-thirds of people with acne report that acne influences their social involvement, and 75% of people report interpersonal issues due to acne. Many people avoid going out or spending time with others when they are suffering from acne flares, which can make them feel uncomfortable and feel like others are looking at their acne during conversations or other interactions. This can lead to anxiety and may continue to be a lifelong issue in some cases, even after the acne flare has improved.

Romantic relationships are another important part of self-image and life satisfaction for many people. Acne has been shown to play a large role in this area as well. The presence of acne has been shown to make people feel as if they have a lower chance of finding a prospective romantic partner, a lower chance of dating or marrying, and a lower chance of being positively thought of by others. In fact, many people with acne report that they have experienced bullying or teasing by peers and relatives because of their acne.

Another important impact of acne on self-image involves the way that people interact with the world around them and the activities that they choose to engage in. When an individual's self-image is negatively changed by acne, it can demotivate them and discourage them from engaging in recreational activities in the broader world. For example, those with acne are less likely to engage in physical activity or exercise. In one study, nearly 10% of schoolchildren reported avoiding swimming and other sports because of embarrassment from their acne. This can also spread into other domains of life, with acne resulting in higher rates of poor school performance and even unemployment in adulthood.

The widespread and significant impact of acne on almost every part of self-worth means that acne is a serious medical condition that deserves attention and treatment in an efficient way. Thankfully, most forms of acne are able to be effectively managed and treated with medications and some lifestyle habit changes. The early treatment of acne before it can impact psychological well-being and self-image is crucial to ensuring health on a physical, mental, and emotional level. In fact, this has prompted health-care professionals and interest societies to advocate for easier access to health care for all adolescents and more acne screening and treatment services in schools, health clinics, and other spaces that adolescents and young adults use.

26. Can having acne lead to depression?

One of the many impacts that acne can have on the emotional and mental state of individuals is causing or worsening depression. In this way, acne can significantly impact the quality of life and well-being of people who suffer from the condition.

Although feeling sad or negative at times is a normal part of life for all people, depression occurs when these feelings are persistent and do not go away. Depression is a mood disorder that is characterized by feelings of sadness, loss of interest in activities, changing appetites, loss of energy or increased fatigue, feelings of guilt or worthlessness, difficulty concentrating, and even thoughts of death or suicide. In those who suffer from depression, these feelings last for longer than two weeks and interfere with their ability to lead normal, healthy lives. Importantly, depression is not a personal failing or the fault of the person suffering from the condition. Depression is a medical condition that involves the brain and is influenced by an individual's thoughts, experiences, and behavior and the external world that an individual lives in. Acne is one of the countless different factors that can contribute to the development of depression or the worsening of preexisting depression.

Although approximately 6% of adults suffer from depression at any moment, and about 16% of people suffer from depression at some point in their lifetime, almost 30% of people who suffer from skin conditions experience depression. Therefore, there is a tremendous link between skin conditions such as acne and the development of mental health issues such as depression. Typically, the worse that the skin condition becomes, the larger the impact that it has on mental health and depression.

In cases of moderate to severe acne, the presence of acne bumps and scars can cause people to isolate themselves and withdraw from social interaction. This withdrawal from social interaction and the outside world can be as simple as reducing involvement in sports or extracurricular activities, or it can be as severe as being scared to even leave the home environment. This level of isolation then serves to increase the risk of developing depression.

In addition, acne can affect self-image to such a significant degree that it can cause lifelong changes in the way that individuals view themselves. This means that people can develop depression from negative thoughts and self-views, even once acne lesions improve and are not as much of an issue. *Dysmorphia* is the medical term for this process where an individual's perception of his or her physical experience becomes disconnected from reality. Dysmorphia from acne and other medical conditions can be a lifelong issue and significantly increases the risk for depression and other mental health issues. In people who suffer from dysmorphia, therapy with a psychologist and even treatment with medications are often needed to overcome the condition.

The link between acne and the development of depression is so strong that many medical professionals recommend the regular use of screening surveys for depression at dermatology appointments. This would allow the medical system to identify people who suffer from acne-related depression as early as possible to get them the appropriate medical and psychological treatment that they need. An effective approach to treating acne-related depression would involve treating both the acne and the depression that has developed.

Unfortunately, mental health issues in many parts of the world, including the United States, are viewed with stigma and negativity. The myth that depression is a choice and indicates a personal failing has remained common, despite evidence that depression involves changes in the function and structure of the brain itself. In fact, 98% of people in one research survey agreed that people with mental illness suffer from stigma and prejudice. Because of this, many people feel embarrassed and ashamed to seek treatment for depression that develops as a result of acne. More than half of the people with mental illnesses, such as depression, never seek treatment for their condition. However, depression can frequently be successfully treated with antidepressants and psychotherapy in those that are able to seek care. Therefore, it is important to encourage people to seek care for depression and to break the stigmas associated with mental health treatment in the United States.

27. Is it okay to pick at acne bumps?

Picking at acne bumps is one of the worst things that someone with acne can do, and it should be avoided as much as possible by people who suffer from acne. Unfortunately, it is also an extremely common habit among those with acne, despite how harmful it can be.

There are a number of reasons why picking at acne bumps is such a common behavior. One of the major reasons is because of the presence of itch, which is known as *pruritis* in medical terms. Itch is a very common symptom that accompanies inflammation and irritation of the skin. This is because the skin contains many nerve receptors that become activated by the presence of pressure and inflammation. When these nerve receptors are activated, they carry a signal from the skin to the brain, which creates the sensation of itch. Itch creates the strong urge to scratch, which can be very challenging to resist in people who suffer from acne.

In addition to itch, the misconception that picking at acne bumps can lead to faster improvement of acne is another common reason why people with acne pick at their skin. While picking at acne bumps can feel gratifying and empowering, it does not help the skin heal faster. In fact, picking acne bumps can cause damage that takes even longer to heal and resolve. Unfortunately, the damage that picking at acne bumps causes often results in permanent scarring, which is why picking at acne bumps is so strongly discouraged.

Although moderate and severe forms of acne can result in permanent scarring even without picking at acne bumps, mild forms of acne tend to resolve on their own and leave no permanent changes to the skin. This is because the body is able to regrow normal skin in the area of the acne once the condition improves. However, when there is picking at the area, it can result in damage that disturbs the surrounding skin and causes the new skin to grow in an abnormal way, resulting in scarring. The scarred skin can be rougher and elevated, or it can be depressed and look different from the surrounding skin. In fact, acne scarring is often just as much of a distressing skin condition as the acne.

In addition to resulting in permanent scarring, picking at acne bumps can also result in an increased risk of skin infections. One of the most important functions of skin is to serve as a barrier between the outside world and the inside of the body. This barrier serves as a wall that keeps out bacteria, viruses, and other organisms that can cause infection and harm the body. When the barrier of the skin is broken by damage, infectious organisms such as bacteria are able to enter the skin and the body, causing infection and harm. By picking at acne bumps, the integrity of the skin can be broken, which increases the risk of infection. Infections of the skin, known as cellulitis, can be painful and result in significant redness, swelling, and discomfort. Antibiotics are often needed to prevent cellulitis from spreading and causing harm.

When picking at acne bumps becomes a regular habit, it can result in the development of other skin conditions in addition to the underlying acne. Picking at the skin can cause the development of nodules, or deep round bumps on the skin, and it causes inflammation, which can result in splotchy skin color. The presence of these nodules as a result of skin picking is labeled as a disease called purigo nodularis. *Purigo* means "itch," and *nodularis* refers to the presence of nodules. Interestingly, these nodules, which are the result of skin picking, can themselves become itchy and cause people to pick their skin even more. It then becomes a self-perpetuating cycle that can cause a lot of skin damage and significant discomfort.

To avoid the harmful behavior of picking at acne bumps, there are a variety of techniques that can be useful. Spot treatment of individual acne bumps can be an effective way of avoiding skin-picking behaviors. In spot treatment, a small amount of topical acne medication is applied on a single acne bump or a small area with a few acne bumps. This allows the medication to work directly on the affected skin, and it allows the person with acne to feel empowered to fix the acne without relying on picking at the acne bumps. In addition, spot treatment can help to reduce the itch that often causes skin picking, which can reduce the chances of skin picking occurring. While spot treatment does not prevent acne bumps from happening in the first place, it can be a helpful resource in the tool kit of people with acne, especially those with itch and discomfort from their acne bumps.

In addition to spot treatment, behavior modification is an important part of avoiding skin picking in acne. Behavior modification refers to the technique of changing behavior by paying attention to the behavior and correcting negative behaviors as soon as the mind becomes aware of it. Since a lot of skin picking occurs mindlessly, it is almost impossible to completely eliminate skin picking. However, by stopping the picking behavior every time upon becoming aware of it, the amount of time spent picking at acne bumps can be significantly reduced.

28. Does anything help make acne less itchy?

The classic form of acne that has whiteheads and blackheads without much redness or irritation does not usually itch on its own. However, if the area becomes inflamed or irritated, it can become very itchy, which can be a huge bother for people with acne.

One of the most common reasons that noninflammatory acne becomes itchy is because of frequent touching and scratching of the area. Many people with acne mindlessly pick at their acne bumps or frequently touch their pimples, which can be very irritating for the skin in that area. When the skin becomes irritated, the process of inflammation occurs and can lead to significant itch.

The process of inflammation in the skin is complex, but one of first steps usually involves the widening of blood vessels to allow for the entrance of inflammatory cells into the skin and underlying tissue. This widening of blood vessels is what is responsible for the red appearance of irritated or inflamed skin. The inflammatory cells that enter the skin from these blood vessels can release chemicals that make the inflammation worse, activating nerves in the skin that then send itch signals to the brain. The activation of these nerves is what is responsible for the horrible itch that can occur in inflamed skin. Unfortunately, once the process of inflammation has started, it can be a self-perpetuating cycle that is hard to break through.

There are a variety of ways to prevent, reduce, and control the amount of itch that people with acne suffer from. The most important of these approaches is prevention, as the process of inflammation and itch can be very challenging to stop once it has started. To prevent acne bumps from itching, building good habits and getting appropriate treatment for acne are essential steps. Habits that can help to prevent acne from becoming irritated and itchy include not touching acne bumps frequently, not picking at acne bumps, and removing dirt, sweat, and other irritating materials by cleaning the face with gentle cleansers. It is also important for the underlying acne to be appropriately treated with medications since poorly controlled acne can develop significant inflammation and itch even without scratching or picking. Overall, prevention through the building of healthy habits and the appropriate treatment of acne is the best way to avoid itch from becoming a major complication of acne.

However, sometimes it is not possible to prevent acne from becoming itchy. This is especially true for people who suffer from inflammatory acne. People with inflammatory acne often have significant redness around the acne, pimples, nodules, and cysts and significant itch in the areas of their breakouts. For the itch in this form of acne, there are a variety of medications that can help. Avoiding scratching the area and continuing treatment of the acne with appropriate medications are still essential, but a number of different additional medications can target the itch, including antihistamines, antibiotics, and even cold compresses.

Antihistamines are one of the most effective anti-itch medications available because they target the chemicals and receptors that inflammatory cells use to cause itch. By using antihistamines, these chemical receptors are blocked, and the nerves responsible for causing the feeling of itchiness are activated less than before. While there are antihistamines that come in oral form, the most appropriate antihistamine medications for acne are usually the topical forms that come in creams, gels, and ointments. These can be applied to areas with significant itch, usually on the face and trunk, and they work rather quickly to reduce itch and provide relief.

In addition, most people with inflammatory acne are recommended to get treatment with oral or topical antibiotics. This is because the overgrowth of normal bacteria on the skin is often responsible for a major part of the inflammation that is seen in inflammatory acne. Since this inflammation leads to the significant itch that can be seen in inflammatory acne, targeting these bacteria is a key step in reducing inflammation and the level of itch that is experienced. Importantly, however, antibiotic medications do not usually directly influence inflammation or reduce itch, so they are only appropriate when bacteria are responsible for contributing to inflammation and itch. Therefore, antibiotics are usually only used in certain cases of acne, such as inflammatory acne.

29. Can you wear makeup with acne?

Many people wonder about whether they are able to wear makeup with acne, and, thankfully, most people with acne are able to safely wear makeup on a regular basis without worsening their acne. However, it is important that people with acne take several steps to make sure that their makeup products and routines are compatible with their skin and do not worsen their acne.

One of the most common sources of acne in relation to makeup is the use of makeup products that cause skin irritation or skin sensitivity. Every person's skin is unique and different; therefore, skin-care products that work well for one individual's skin may cause significant irritation and discomfort for another person's skin. Therefore, people who wear makeup and use a variety of skin-care products should always be on the lookout to see whether there is an association between the products that they use and sensitivity in their skin. If they find that a skin-care or makeup product causes their skin to become sensitive, irritated, or have an acne breakout, they should stop using that product and find a better alternative. This is an especially important point with makeup products that include multiple fragrances, natural extracts, or essential oils, as these chemicals can trigger sensitivities in some people. Additionally, many makeup products share multiple ingredients and components, so once a skin sensitivity is identified, future makeup products should be checked for those components before they are used.

A popular movement in the world of makeup is the increasing use of makeup ingredients that are gentler on the skin and less likely to trigger the appearance of acne. These ingredients are often labeled as *noncomedogenic*, which means that they are less likely to cause whiteheads or blackheads. Although noncomedogenic ingredients and makeups are not perfect and do not guarantee that they will not cause skin sensitivity and acne breakouts, they can reduce the risk of makeup contributing to the worsening of acne.

Another common issue with makeup for people who have acne is the lack of a healthy and effective makeup removal routine. While most makeups are made to be compatible with skin pores and minimize the risk of developing acne, leaving makeup on the skin for long periods of time can lead to plugged skin pores and the development of acne. Therefore, it is important to wash off makeup before sleep or after long periods of time so that the skin is able to function and shed normally. This is also important for makeup around the eye, which can often be missed or forgotten during cleansing routines.

While cleaning makeup from the face is a good way of reducing the risk of acne from makeup, it is important to use gentle cleansers and not cleanse the skin too intensely. Frequent skin washing, using rough chemical cleansers, or physically rubbing the skin too hard can all contribute to skin dryness, irritation, and acne breakouts. Therefore, the best way to keep skin healthy while wearing makeup is to only use gentle cleansers a couple of times a day to effectively wash off makeup and keep the skin hydrated. Most people prefer to wash their face once in the morning after waking and once in the evening before sleeping. This balanced approach to skin care allows the skin to remain clean while avoiding the negative impacts of overwashing.

With acne, it is also important to apply makeup gently to avoid irritation of the skin. Many people use makeup applicators and brushes, which can vary a lot in the pressure and texture applied to the skin. Brushing or applying makeup too heavily can scratch the skin or cause irritation, dryness, or discomfort, which can all lead to the start or worsening of acne.

In addition to gently applying makeup, frequently cleaning and changing out makeup tools is another important step to ensure that makeup is working with the skin and not contributing to the development of acne. Many people fall into a routine of using the same makeup application tools and brushes without changing or cleaning them effectively. This can result in the application of dirt, old skin oils, and dead skin cell debris onto the skin, resulting in the plugging of follicles and development of acne. This is also a common problem for people who frequently share makeup with friends and family. Therefore, the risk of developing acne from makeup can be reduced by frequently cleaning or changing out makeup tools and by avoiding sharing these tools with other people.

Finally, despite taking all of these steps to promote healthy skin while using makeup, acne can still happen. If that is the case, it is important to treat the acne once it happens. While stopping possible suspect makeups can be an important step in helping acne heal, the use of acne medications can help make the process more effective and timely. In fact, with the help of acne medications, millions of people are able to happily and successfully wear makeup while experiencing acne breakouts without making their acne worse.

30. How can I change my skin-care routine to help with acne?

Some of the most powerful tools for a healthy life are healthy habits and routines, and skin care is no exception. The ability of a healthy skin-care routine to help improve acne is impressive, especially when combined with an appropriate medication regimen. As part of a healthy skin-care routine, there are several steps that are essential for promoting healthy skin and improving acne.

The frequency and timing of skin washing is one of the most important parts of a healthy skin-care routine. This is because there needs to be a fine balance between keeping the skin clean without causing it to become too dried out or irritated. Therefore, most dermatologists recommend gently washing the face about two times a day, usually in the morning after waking and in the evening prior to sleeping. In addition, since sweating can be irritating to the skin, washing the skin lightly after exercise can be helpful to cleanse away sweat and different materials.

In addition to the frequency and timing of skin washing, the way that the skin is washed is important. Most dermatologists recommend washing the skin with water or gentle cleansers that are applied lightly on the skin with the fingertips. The use of fingertips rather than brushes, towels, or other fabrics is important because material other than the fingertips can cause irritation of the skin. Of course, it is still important to always use gentle cleansers and chemicals to avoid excessive skin drying and irritation of the skin. Also, while many brands and companies market products such as micellar water or ultrapure water at high price tags, these are largely unnecessary as long as clean tap or filtered water is available.

Another important component of a healthy skin-care routine for acne is the use of appropriately warmed water. Many people develop a tendency to shower or wash the face with hot water, which can be dehydrating and irritating for the skin. This increases the risk of acne and can cause discomfort, itch, and redness. Therefore, using lukewarm water can reduce the risk of irritation and help to improve acne as part of an overall skin-care routine.

Interestingly, the order of product use for skin care also plays an important role for all people, including those with acne. It is especially important for those with acne because they require additional products, such as acne medications, as part of their skin-care routines in the morning and evening. Most people should apply lukewarm water or a gentle cleanser to their skin first to clean away dirt and dead skin. Then, toner, serums, and eye creams should be applied and allowed to settle on the skin. After that, spot treatments or acne medications can be put on the skin. Moisturizers should be placed on last as well as most physical sunscreen lotions. Importantly however, there are some sunscreen lotions that use chemicals and are referred to as chemical sunscreens; these chemical sunscreens need to be placed on the skin first rather than last.

Additionally, even the timing with which acne medications are applied can make a difference. Many acne washes, including those with the most popular medical ingredient, benzoyl peroxide, can react with other medications on the skin and inactivate them. Therefore, benzoyl peroxide should not be applied on the skin at the same time as other topical acne treatments, such as antibiotics or retinoid medications. In these cases, the benzoyl peroxide can be applied at a different time of the day, or it can be applied and washed off, with application of the other medications later on. Spreading out the timing of benzoyl peroxide and other topi-cal acne medications ensures that those additional medications are not inactivated.

Finally, one of the most counterintuitive changes that can be made to a skin-care routine is to stop changing the skin-care routine so frequently. Many people who suffer from acne can understandably become frustrated in trying to find a skin-care routine that will help improve their acne. Because of this frustration, people can cycle through different skin-care routines, various skin-care products, and different medication regimens rather quickly in the hope that they will find something that works for them. However, most skin-care routines and even most acne medication treatment regimens take time to work and begin to affect the skin. In fact, even people who begin acne medication treatment directed by a dermatologist will not experience improvement of their acne for several weeks, until the medications have had time to significantly influence the skin. Thus, it makes sense that frequent changes in skin-care routines and cycling through different products without giving them time to show their impact can be a very frustrating and ultimately futile experience. There-fore, when making changes to a skin-care routine, time should be given to see how the skin is affected over the course of weeks and months rather than hours and days.

31. What other lifestyle modifications can help with acne?

While acne is a medical condition of the skin that requires medical treat-ment to improve in a timely and effective way, there are a variety of life-style changes that can help to improve acne and reduce the number of acne breakouts that happen. In fact, lifestyle changes are a powerful tool that can enhance the effectiveness of an acne treatment regimen and allow for better skin over the long term.

One of the most important lifestyle modifications for all people, espe-cially those who suffer from acne, is protecting the skin against exposure to the sun. This is because the light from the sun is actually a form of ultraviolet (UV) radiation, which is a powerful kind of energy. While sunlight is extraordinary in illuminating the world and giving energy to plants and life on earth, the energy in sunlight can damage skin in a sub-tle way that only becomes apparent over long periods of time. In fact, exposure to sunlight is one of the major contributors to the development of wrinkles, the aging of skin, and even the development of most forms of skin cancer. This is especially a big problem when skin becomes sunburnt from too much sun exposure at once, which can lead to redness, irritation, and even blistering.

For people with acne, as well as those who do not have acne, it is important to wear sun protection when outside, especially during peak sunlight hours. Sun protection can include clothing that covers exposed areas of skin, such as a hat or long pants and long-sleeved shirts, or it can involve the use of a sunscreen lotion or makeup that includes chemicals that layer on top of the skin and prevent sunlight from reaching into the skin itself. These forms of sunscreen are categorized by a system called SPF, which stands for sun protection factor. The SPF of a sunscreen or sun-protectant clothing is a measure of how much solar energy is needed to cause a sunburn on the protected skin. For example, all people are recommended to use sun protection with a rating of SPF 30 or higher when being exposed to sunlight. An SPF 30 sunscreen protects the skin so that it will take 30 times more solar energy to cause a sunburn on the protected skin than unprotected skin. This allows people to enjoy more time outside while reducing the damage that sunlight causes on their skin. Importantly, however, the skin can still become damaged by sunlight over a long enough period of time, even when using sun protection.

Many people wonder whether it is worth purchasing and using sun protection with higher SPF ratings; many sunscreen lotions go up to SPF 60 or SPF 100. While increasing SPF ratings means that the sun protection is more effective, there is a point where the increasing level of protection is not as meaningful. For example, the recommended minimum of SPF 30 already blocks 97% of UVB rays, while SPF 50 blocks 98% and SPF 100 blocks 99%. As the SPF increases, the cost of the sunscreen usually increases significantly, so it can become costly to use enough of the higher SPF sunscreen to fully cover the skin and to consistently reapply the sunscreen every two hours as recommended. Therefore, it is better to buy and use an SPF 30 correctly than to buy an SPF 50 or SPF 100 sunscreen and not be able to use enough to adequately protect the skin. In addition to using sunscreen, avoiding tanning beds and other forms of artificial UV light exposure is very important for taking care of the health of the skin.

Many of the other lifestyle modifications that are recommended for improving acne are often recommended for improving overall health as well. For example, reducing stress can play a significant role in improving acne in some people by reducing the amount of stress hormones in the body, which can cause acne flares. In addition to improving acne, lowering stress levels can improve the health of the entire body, including the brain and the heart.

Alongside lowering stress levels, ensuring high-quality sleep can have a significant impact on overall health and well-being in addition to improving the appearance and health of the skin. During sleep, the skin and other organs of the body have time to restore, recover, and reinvigorate, and this process is an essential and required part of every person's life. Therefore, prioritizing healthy sleep habits is a key part of a healthy lifestyle and can make a big difference in improving the quality of the skin.

Another large lifestyle factor that can have a big difference for people who suffer from acne is diet. Since food is closely linked with the hormone balance in the body, reducing the amount of high-sugar foods in the diet and prioritizing healthy foods can improve the appearance of acne and reduce the number of acne breakouts that occur. Some people are able to identify foods that are triggers for acne outbreaks in their skin, and avoiding these triggers is another important part of changing diet to improve acne. Importantly, all dietary changes should be done with moderation, and significant dietary changes should be done with the assistance of a health-care provider or registered dietitian. This is because it is important to ensure that a person's diet is well rounded and able to provide all of the necessary nutrients for the body to function correctly.

While lifestyle modifications can have a significant impact on improving acne and reducing the number of acne breakouts, they are not a replacement for medications in the treatment of acne. In fact, lifestyle modifications are most effective when they are combined with an effective acne medication regimen. Together, medical treatment and lifestyle modification are the most effective way of treating and managing acne over the long term.

32. What support resources are available for people with acne?

On the surface, acne may seem like a mild condition because it is not life-threatening on its own and it is so tremendously common. However, the emotional and psychological impact that it can have on individuals is tremendous and can vary significantly from one person to another. Thankfully, there are a number of support resources that exist for people who suffer from acne.

One of the most important support resources for people with acne is the health-care workforce. There are many general physicians, dermatologists, nurse practitioners, physician assistants, and skin-care experts who are trained in the treatment of acne and can provide evidence-based advice and guidance for those who suffer from acne. Doctors and many nurse practitioners and physician assistants are the people who are able to write prescriptions for acne medications, so building a medical relationship with a health-care provider is an important part of treating acne. Oftentimes, cost and insurance coverage can be the largest barrier preventing people from getting medical care, and in these situations, there are a variety of options, including paying a reduced out-of-pocket rate, utilizing a student or free city health clinic, or applying for government-sponsored health insurance, which includes Medicare and Medicaid. In addition, medical schools and universities sometimes offer free or reduced-cost clinics where people without insurance can get access to health care.

In addition to the health-care system, the American Academy of Dermatology (AAD) is one of the best resources for information for people who suffer from any skin condition, including acne. The AAD is the professional group that represents most dermatologists in the United States, and they have an extensive website that offers information on almost all acne topics. The information that their website provides is vetted to be factual and easy to understand. Unfortunately, the quality of information on the Internet can vary widely, so using the AAD as a primary source of information regarding acne ensures that it is high quality and trustworthy.

Another valuable support resource for people who suffer from acne includes acne support groups and classes, which can help comfort people with acne and educate them regarding their skin condition. Acne support groups are usually sponsored by health-care organizations, perhaps in a surrounding town or city, so reaching out to local hospitals, health clinics, or health-care centers can be an effective way of finding and connecting with acne support groups. With the expansion of access to the Internet, some acne support groups have recently become available online as well, in the form of forums and online meetings. Video conferencing technology, for example, has greatly extended the range and accessibility of medical support groups in recent years.

The emotional and psychological burden of acne can often be troubling for people who suffer from the condition. In these situations, it can be tremendously helpful to seek psychological counseling or therapy with the assistance of a mental health therapist or psychologist. The role of these therapists often involves training individuals to reinforce healthy and positive mental patterns of thought while addressing and resolving negative thoughts and habits. In some cases, people with depression or anxiety from their acne can benefit from psychiatric care that involves the use of medications in addition to mental health counseling to improve mental health. Although it can feel isolating and sometimes even embarrassing to suffer from mental health issues, mental health problems are very common, and most people can get a huge benefit from getting psychologic or psychiatric care. The mind and psychological health of a person are just like any other organ of the body and require treatment and attention in the same way that other organs do.

Finally, acne can be so emotionally distressing to some people that they start to have thoughts of hurting themselves or even committing suicide. Having these thoughts of self-harm is an important red flag that should prompt seeking care with a doctor as soon as possible. In urgent situations, going to the nearest emergency department is a good option. If that is not possible, then the National Suicide Prevention Hotline is a resource that allows those who are contemplating suicide to get help quickly. The National Suicide Prevention Hotline can be reached at 1-800-273-8255 at any time by any person in the United States. It can be scary or troubling to experience thoughts of self-harm or suicide, but seeking help when such thoughts occur is very important.

Acne Treatments

33. When does acne need to be treated by a doctor?

The simple answer is that acne should be treated by a doctor when it becomes bothersome to the person suffering from it. Although acne is almost a universal human experience because of how common it is, many people suffer from very mild acne that does not bother them or cause any disruption in their appearance or day-to-day life. Many people with this mild type of acne prefer to avoid any treatment of their acne, choosing instead to let the rare acne bump come and go on its own. Others might use spot treatments only when they experience an acne bump and otherwise prefer not to keep up with a regular skin-care regimen.

However, a good proportion of other people experience an acne that is frequent or widespread enough to bother them. In these situations, getting treatment for acne is completely appropriate. In fact, most dermatologists would say that there is never a wrong time to seek treatment for acne. Some people with this mild to moderate form of acne prefer to try to self-treat first by using acne products that are available over the counter, while the rest prefer to start off by pursuing the assistance of a general physician or a dermatologist.

For those that prefer to self-treat their acne with over-the-counter medications, there are some indicators or signs that they should get treatment for their acne by a doctor. One of the biggest signs is trying over-the-counter acne products and not seeing effective results. Although all acne regimens take several weeks to work, if a skin-care routine using acne medications is not working effectively by that time, it is appropriate to consult a dermatologist or other physician for assistance and guidance. This is particularly important to avoid delaying the improvement of the skin and the resolution of acne, especially because acne is temporary when treated early but can cause permanent scarring if left untreated.

Another common sign that it is time to get acne treatment from a doctor is the worsening or changing of acne. Many people suffer from mild acne and choose not to pursue treatment for it. However, when their acne becomes more severe and symptoms worsen, it is appropriate to seek medical care. Additionally, if acne begins to change color, leak fluid, or become more tender and painful than usual, getting help from a doctor is completely appropriate. Sometimes, acne can become infected with bacteria and other microorganisms, and in these situations, getting medical care and antibiotics quickly is important. People who are worried about an infection of their acne are encouraged to make a same-week appointment with their primary care doctor or to seek a walk-in visit at the local urgent care.

In addition, the logistics of health care in the United States is an important consideration for some people when choosing when to get medical treatment for acne. Many people in the United States are dependent on their family or employer for health insurance coverage, and seeking care from a physician while covered under health insurance is a smart move. For example, many people make multiple appointments with different specialists to get their regular checkups all sorted out before they leave a job with medical insurance or grow too old to be a part of their parent's health insurance. This allows them to get as much medical care as possible before they lose insurance coverage. Also, many health insurance plans require people to pay a certain amount of money before the health insurance plan starts to cover the cost of health care. In these situations, people who have already paid that required minimum amount may want to maximize the amount of health care that they get that year since their health insurance will cover the majority of it.

Ultimately, however, the most important takeaway is that there is never a wrong time to get treatment for acne with the help of a physician. Acne affects each person uniquely, and getting treatment is just as appropriate for the mildest acne as it is for the most severe acne. It is always better to get medical treatment early than it is to delay and get medical treatment too late, especially because acne can be scarring when it is left untreated.

In addition, seeing a physician for acne does not have to be a long-term commitment. Many people meet with a dermatologist for an initial consultation, get the advice and his or her medical opinion, and then make a decision later regarding whether to pursue medical treatment of their acne. Speaking with a dermatologist or other physician can be immensely helpful for answering questions, getting educated advice, and having a trained professional share their experience and knowledge.

Unfortunately, one of the most common barriers that prevents people from pursuing medical treatment of their acne with a physician is embarrassment or self-consciousness regarding their acne. Some people feel as if their acne is not bad enough to warrant medical care, and they feel as if they will be ridiculed for seeking treatment, especially if their acne is mild. Others do not want to bring attention to their acne, and they believe that the experience of seeing a doctor and being examined might be humiliating. While seeing a physician can be an involved and personal process, physicians are trained to provide respectful and considerate care to all people. Dermatologists also understand the impact that acne can have on each individual regardless of how mild or severe the condition is. Therefore, it is important to overcome these barriers to care when they occur and to not let them prevent getting effective treatment for acne early on.

34. What types of doctors are trained to treat acne?

The structure and organization of the health-care system can be a whirlwind of confusion at times. This is especially true when trying to decide what type of health-care professional to get help from to treat acne. There are a wide variety of health-care specialties, including nursing, nurse practitioners, physician assistants, and physicians. In addition, even among physicians, there are a variety of specialties that exist, including family medicine and dermatology. Beyond that, there are a large number of different practice environments that health-care providers work in, including clinics, hospitals, universities, and other organizations. Therefore, understanding each of those roles and locations can be helpful in getting treatment for acne from trained and appropriate professionals.

Understanding the different health-care roles and their level of training is a good place to start. The most extensively trained health-care providers are physicians. Physicians can be referred to under a number of titles, including physician, doctor, surgeon, MD, and DO. Despite these many terms, all physicians go to medical school and complete a residency training program where they learn to manage a wide range of medical conditions, including rare and complex diseases.

In addition, physicians are able to specialize their training during their residency program. Because of this, physicians are often referred to by their chosen specialty. Physicians that specialize in the skin are called dermatologists, while those that choose to pursue general practice are referred to as family physicians or internal medicine doctors. Interestingly, some physicians decide to become subspecialists, where they narrow their focus even more. For example, a dermatologist may become a cosmetic dermatologist by pursuing extra training on cosmetic procedures or a pediatric dermatologist by working primarily with children.

Among the physician specialties that treat acne, dermatology and family medicine are the two most common. Family medicine and internal medicine doctors are the generalist physicians that manage all types of diseases affecting every part of the body. While they are able to treat the mild to moderate forms of acne, severe acne and acne with red flags should be referred to dermatologists. Dermatologist are specifically trained in skin conditions and are the experts in treating acne and other diseases of the skin. They are able to tackle complex cases of acne and use specialized medications that require close monitoring. In addition to general physicians and dermatologists, other clinicians are frequently involved in treating acne. Pediatricians are physicians who care for children, and since many adolescents experience acne, pediatricians are commonly involved in treating the condition. Obstetrics and gynecology (OBGYN) doctors are often asked to treat acne by their female patients, especially when there is a hormonal component to their acne flares. For people with severe acne scarring, sometimes plastic surgeons can be involved in treatment as well. While each of these fields has a specific focus, they are all equipped to handle most components of treating basic acne.

Although less trained than physicians, nurse practitioners and physician assistants are another form of health-care provider that can provide treatment for acne. Nurse practitioners and physician assistants are trained to diagnose and manage basic and common medical conditions with direct supervision from a physician. Many doctor's offices and health-care systems use teams of nurse practitioners and physician assistants to provide care to patients for simple visits, such as follow-up checks, while utilizing physicians for complex cases and initial visits. Many dermatology offices employ nurse practitioners and physician assistants to manage common skin conditions, such as mild acne, eczema, and dermatitis. While this practice is appropriate, it is important to make sure that there is oversight from a physician who is able to step in and assist if there are challenges or complications.

In addition to the different kinds of health-care providers, there are also various health-care settings where the treatment of acne can be received. Many people prefer to go to a doctor's office or dermatology clinic for treatment of their acne. Many of these offices belong to a local physician or are part of a small chain of practices. These are often preferred by people who like small businesses or forming a personal relationship with their physician. Alternatively, many other physicians work for health-care systems, large hospitals, or university health networks. These larger systems are often more compatible with insurance companies and can offer access to very highly trained specialists that focus on specific rare and complex conditions. While the practice setting is largely up to the personal preference of each individual, people who suffer from complex acne often require a referral to a hospital or university clinic to get specialized care.

Despite how complex the structure of the medical system might be in the United States, it is important not to let it become a barrier to getting treatment for acne. Making an appointment with a family physician or a dermatologist is always a good place to start, and most physicians are able to make referrals to other more appropriate health-care providers when appropriate. The most important step is making the initial appointment and attending it.

35. What is benzoyl peroxide? How does it help acne?

Benzoyl peroxide is one of the most common acne medications used worldwide. There are countless cleansers, face washes, creams, and foams that use benzoyl peroxide as their main ingredient to combat acne. In fact, almost every recommended acne regimen uses benzoyl peroxide in one form or another because of its ability to cleanse the skin and kill bacteria. While companies such as CeraVe, PanOxyl, Differin, La Roche-Posay, and Neutrogena all sell their own cleansers under unique brand names, they share the same essential ingredient known as benzoyl peroxide.

At its simplest, benzoyl peroxide is a chemical that has a mild bleaching effect. This chemical bleaching effect is largely responsible for the high efficacy that it has when applied on skin with acne. In fact, the bleaching effect of benzoyl peroxide has been shown to help improve acne by three separate mechanisms of action that act on the skin to help normalize it.

The first major way that benzoyl peroxide works on the skin involves its action as a sebostatic agent. The term *sebostatic* refers to the ability of benzoyl peroxide to slow or stop the production of sebum, or skin oil, on the surface of the skin. While these natural skin oils are essential in regulating the health and moisture of skin, they can contribute to acne when their production is significantly increased above normal levels. Therefore, in skin affected by acne, the effect of benzoyl peroxide to slow down and reduce the production of excess sebum helps to improve the health of the skin and reduce the severity of acne.

Another major way that benzoyl peroxide contributes to improving acne is by acting as a comedolytic agent. Comedones are the skin pores that become clogged with skin oils and dead skin cells to form the classic bumps of acne. The term *comedolytic* refers to the ability of benzoyl peroxide to break apart these clogged skin pores or acne bumps and help the skin become normal. While there are many chemicals that act as comedolytic agents, including salicylic acid and azelaic acid, benzoyl peroxide is by far the most studied and most popular comedolytic ingredient used in acne medications. The frequent use of benzoyl peroxide also helps to prevent the formation of comedones in the first place.

Finally, the ability of benzoyl peroxide to kill bacteria and act as an antibiotic agent is another effect that makes it such a power and effective tool in treating acne. The bleaching effect of benzoyl peroxide allows it to break apart bacteria and control the overgrowth of bacteria on the skin of people with acne. In fact, this is a tremendously useful capability of benzoyl peroxide because it allows the chemical to combine its effectiveness with other antibiotics to target bacteria in multiple ways and reduce the chance of bacterial resistance. This is why benzoyl peroxide is commonly prescribed whenever antibiotics are used in treating acne.

Some studies have shown that benzoyl peroxide may also play an anti-inflammatory role in the skin by reducing the amount of inflammatory chemicals released by the immune system. This effect is less understood than the others that benzoyl peroxide is known for. However, it is definitely possible that this anti-inflammatory effect could have a beneficial impact on acne.

Although it is so frequently used, benzoyl peroxide does have some side effects that are important to be aware of. Since it has a bleaching effect, it can be irritating to the skin and result in mild redness, a burning sensation, or skin sensitivity. This is why most dermatologists recommend slowly building up a daily skin-care routine with benzoyl peroxide by applying it just once a day or every other day for several days or weeks before going up to using it twice a day every day.

In addition, the bleaching effect of benzoyl peroxide means that it can sometimes react with other chemicals and medications to inactivate them. This interaction is most commonly seen between benzoyl peroxide and retinoid medications that are also frequently prescribed. Therefore, the recommendation is to apply benzoyl peroxide on its own and then apply other medications and skin-care products separately at a later time.

The bleaching power of benzoyl peroxide may also affect fabrics. It can cause whitening of clothing or bedsheets if it is spilled or the face is not fully washed after use. Therefore, most dermatologists recommend carefully washing the face after using benzoyl peroxide and avoiding wearing delicate or expensive clothing while using the medication.

Despite these minor side effects, benzoyl peroxide remains one of the most frequently prescribed and used medications in the treatment of acne. It is largely a safe medication with tens to hundreds of millions of people having used it. Therefore, it should continue to be a key part of most acne skin-care routines.

36. Can antibiotics help with treating acne?

Although antibiotics are rarely used alone in the treatment of acne, they are a powerful tool in a multipronged approach to treating acne. Acne is not caused by just bacteria, but the overgrowth of bacteria on the skin can be a contributing factor in the development and worsening of acne. Therefore, medications that target this bacterial overgrowth and help to normalize the number of bacteria on the skin can be useful in the treatment of acne. This is especially true in inflammatory acne and moderate to severe acne, where the role of bacteria is thought to have greater importance than in mild classic acne. Therefore, antibiotics are often prescribed in treating these more severe forms of acne.

The antibiotics that are used in the treatment of acne come in a variety of different forms. Topical antibiotics are commonly used for the beneficial effect of antibiotics on controlling the population of bacteria on the skin while avoiding the side effects of oral antibiotics. However, when acne is widespread or more severe, oral antibiotics are commonly used as well.

The most commonly used antibiotics in the treatment of acne include doxycycline, minocycline, clindamycin, and erythromycin. To avoid the development of resistance against these medications, the use of antibiotics is usually paired with the application of medications such as benzoyl peroxide to simultaneously target bacteria through different mechanisms of action. This allows bacteria to be attacked in multiple ways and helps to avoid a situation where bacteria might survive with a resistance to the antibiotic.

Doxycycline and minocycline are members of a class of antibiotics called tetracyclines. *Tetracycline* is a term that describes the shape of this class of antibiotics, which features four chemical rings attached to each other. Tetracyclines are powerful inhibitors of protein synthesis in bacteria, which stops bacteria from being able to produce the proteins that they need to grow and survive. This allows them to serve as potent antibiotics that help control the population of bacteria on the skin.

On the other hand, the other commonly used antibiotics, clindamycin and erythromycin, are members of the antibiotic class known as macrolides. The macrolide class of antibiotics share a similar shape, which includes a large ring that has more than a dozen components. Macrolides work in a similar way as tetracyclines by blocking the synthesis of proteins in bacterial cells. However, they target a different part of the protein synthesis process. Interestingly, it has been observed that macrolides can be transported to the site of bacteria by the cells of the immune system, allowing them to target bacteria more effectively.

While these groups of antibiotics are generally safe and well tolerated by most people, there are a variety of side effects that antibiotics can have on people. Oral doxycycline, for example, is known for causing irritation of the esophagus, which is the swallowing tube of the throat. Therefore, most dermatologists recommend drinking a glass of water with doxycycline pills and not lying down for thirty minutes to an hour after taking the medication. In addition, medications such as minocycline can sometimes give a very subtle blue tint to skin and nails when taken over the course of decades. While this is a concerning side effect, it is relatively rare and only occurs after a very long period of use.

Despite these side effects, antibiotics are generally safe and are commonly used in the treatment of acne, especially in moderate to severe cases. For people with acne that features large red bumps or significant inflammation, antibiotics can make a dramatic impact on acne within weeks.

37. How do topical retinoids help with acne?

Retinoids are the cornerstone of acne treatment. In fact, they are the gold standard treatment for almost all cases of acne. While retinoids come in many different forms, such as topical and oral, and various structures, such as retinol, adapalene, and isotretinoin, they all fundamentally work in a similar way.

Retinoids are a group of medications that are based on the structure of vitamin A. Although there are various different retinoids, all of these numerous forms share the same fundamental structure. This similarity with vitamin A allows retinoids to have the ability to influence the function of the skin and, ultimately, help improve acne.

Although the mechanism of action of topical retinoids is quite complex, the fundamental action of retinoids is to act on the receptors of skin cells to change the behavior and function of the skin. Retinoids help to regulate the skin and normalize the way that skin cells function. This is especially important in skin with acne, where functionality is abnormal.

These effects of retinoids are mediated through retinoic acid, which is the final chemical that most retinoids are converted into in the body. Retinoic acid binds to one of the receptors attached on a cell's DNA to change the transcription of genes in the body. This allows retinoids to control which genes are expressed and the degree of their expression, thereby allowing them to control the behavior and action of the body's cells. In fact, retinoids act on a variety of cells through this mechanism, including skin cells, red blood cells, and even the cells of the body's immune system. Interestingly, retinoids have been shown to play a strong anti-inflammatory role in the body as well.

In addition, retinoids can help to break apart comedones, which are the blocked skin pores that are responsible for acne. Therefore, retinoids are known as comedolytic agents. This means that retinoids can not only help to prevent future acne bumps from appearing but also help to improve and resolve current acne blackheads and whiteheads.

Although retinoids come in oral forms, these are usually reserved for moderate to severe forms of acne that can result in severe scarring if not treated immediately. For mild to moderate acne, topical retinoids are preferred because they have fewer side effects and do not significantly affect other organs in the body, such as the liver. In addition, topical retinoids come in different forms, such as creams, gels, and serums, which can be easier to fit into a daily skin-care routine. In fact, most retinoids only require one application a day to be maximally effective.

Interestingly, the effectiveness of topical retinoids is not limited to the treatment of acne. In fact, retinoids have been shown to help reduce the appearance of wrinkles on the skin and to help work as an antiaging medication for the skin. Indeed, retinoids are one of the only medications that have been scientifically proven to have cosmetic antiaging effects on the skin.

Although retinoids are extremely effective in the treatment of acne and skin aging, they are not perfect medications. Topical retinoids are safer and have fewer side effects than oral retinoids, but they still come with important caveats. Topical retinoids make the skin sensitive to sunlight, so it is important to apply topical retinoids in the evening or at nighttime. In addition, it is important to regularly use sunscreen when getting sun exposure to avoid skin irritation and sensitivity. Finally, many people experience a flare in their acne and a temporary worsening of their skin when first starting topical retinoids. Because of this, most dermatologists recommend starting with a lower percentage retinoid cream or serum and working up to a higher potency. In addition, most dermatologists encourage people to start using retinoids once a day only a few days a week before building up to every other day and finally every day. By taking a slow and progressive approach to incorporating retinoids into a daily skin-care routine, the initial flaring and worsening of acne can be reduced, and the transition into using retinoids regularly can be made more natural and easier to tolerate.

38. What is isotretinoin (Accutane)?

While retinoids come in a variety of forms, including topical and oral, the effectiveness of these various forms of retinoids are not the same. In fact, the oral retinoids, such as isotretinoin, are far more potent and have a more powerful influence on the skin than the topical forms, such as adapalene and retinol.

Due to this increased effectiveness, isotretinoin, which is also known by the brand name Accutane, is frequently prescribed as the gold standard therapy for the treatment of severe acne or acne where scarring is a significant risk. However, the price of isotretinoin's effectiveness is the presence of multiple significant side effects, including temporary injury to the liver and risks to developing fetuses. Therefore, the use of isotretinoin comes with significant caveats, including the need for regular blood testing to monitor organ function and the use of contraception to prevent pregnancy while using the medication. However, as long as these safety precautions are taken, isotretinoin is generally a safe and extremely effective medication for the treatment of acne.

Isotretinoin shares the same mechanism of action as other retinoids, which includes binding to receptors in the body's cells and changing the behavior and functioning of those cells. Accutane can even decrease the size of the sebaceous glands in the skin throughout the entire body, reducing the presence of excess oil and preventing the blockage of skin pores throughout the whole body surface area. By controlling sebum production, acne can be reduced and prevented.

Although many people use topical retinoids and face washes like benzoyl peroxide on a daily basis over a long period of time, such as years or even an entire lifetime, isotretinoin is a temporary medication. In fact, most people only require several months of therapy to experience significant improvement of their severe acne. In these people, isotretinoin is taken under close supervision until a total cumulative dose is completed, then they are transitioned off isotretinoin to topical retinoids and other topical acne medications that can be continued long term. Recent research has shown that slightly longer courses of isotretinoin may be more effective at reducing the recurrence of severe acne, but acne treatment courses with isotretinoin are usually not more than six months and almost never more than a year. This helps to prevent side effects and allows people to transition to an easier routine that does not require frequent blood checks or stringent contraception use.

While isotretinoin is a tremendously effective medication and can be safely used under the supervision of a trained dermatologist or other physician, there are a variety of side effects that it can have, which range from common to very rare in frequency. Commonly, people who begin treatment with isotretinoin experience an initial worsening of their acne. These people often describe their acne as the worst that it has ever been during the first couple of weeks of starting isotretinoin. In some people, this acne flare can be severe enough to cause fevers, bone aches, and significant discomfort, which is a condition referred to as *acne fulminans*. In addition, some people can experience headaches, dry eyes, eye irritation, nose bleeds, temporary liver injury, dry skin, itch, and joint pain. Very rarely, changes in mental health, such as depression, anxiety, or even thoughts of suicide and self-harm can occur, especially in younger people. Therefore, careful monitoring and frequent check-ins with a physician are very important while on isotretinoin. Despite these significant side effects, however, most people are able to tolerate isotretinoin without much difficulty.

One of the most important things to consider while on isotretinoin is the importance of contraception use. Because isotretinoin can cause birth defects in the babies of mothers who are on the medication, there is a legal requirement for all people on isotretinoin to register with the iPLEDGE system in the United States, which mandates the use of two forms of contraception, or birth control. Although men, as well as women of nonchildbearing ages, do not have to answer questions each month for the iPLEDGE system, women of reproductive age are required to do so in addition to providing negative pregnancy tests and using at least two forms of contraception at all times. These forms of contraception include abstinence, condom use, oral contraceptives, and IUDs, among others. While isotretinoin can be tremendously effective, these requirements can be quite burdensome and make taking the medication regularly and safely a challenge for many people.

Interestingly, in addition to the use of isotretinoin as an acne medication, it has also been shown to be effective in the treatment of multiple other skin conditions, including hidradenitis suppurativa. Hidradenitis suppurative is similar to acne because it affects areas of the body that are rich in sebaceous glands. Isotretinoin has also been used for other conditions, such as rosacea, when they do not respond to conventional therapies. Therefore, isotretinoin is a versatile and effective drug that is used for a variety of skin conditions. While it carries many side effects, it is possible to use it safely with the help of a well-trained physician, and there are millions of people throughout the world who have accomplished fantastic control of their acne through the use of isotretinoin.

39. What is the iPLEDGE program?

Isotretinoin is a powerful medication that can improve acne more than nearly any other medication known to the medical community. While this makes isotretinoin a wonderful tool for people who suffer from acne, it comes with a significant impact on the body that requires careful monitoring under the supervision of a trained physician, preferably a dermatologist.

Although isotretinoin is able to improve even the most severe acne over the course of several months, it has a variety of potential side effects that need to be taken very seriously. These side effects include injuring the liver, eyes, and other organs of the body. Importantly, isotretinoin can negatively affect pregnancies by causing severe birth defects in developing fetuses. To reduce the risk of these side effects, isotretinoin is a carefully monitored prescription drug that requires the expertise of a trained physician to prescribe. However, the risk of birth defects is serious enough that an additional layer of protection is imposed by the federal government. This additional system is known as the iPLEDGE system.

The iPLEDGE system is a nationwide program run by the U.S. Food and Drug Administration (FDA) with the goal of regulating isotretinoin and minimizing the risk of serious birth defects during pregnancy. The iPLEDGE program has been in existence since 2006, and it has grown in complexity over the years. It was developed as a response to the high rate of pregnancy among patients who were taking isotretinoin and experiencing serious birth defects in their newborns. Unfortunately, prior to the iPLEDGE system, thousands of individuals became pregnant while on the medication and went on to experience abortion, miscarriage, or serious birth defects.

In the early 2000s, the System to Manage Accutane-Related Teratogenicity (SMART) program was developed as an attempt to reduce the rate of birth defects and negative pregnancy outcomes associated with isotretinoin. However, the SMART program was not a requirement of using isotretinoin; participation was voluntary, which meant that the rate of physicians and patients using the system was very low, and there was a minimal impact on the overall rate of birth defects. Therefore, the iPLEDGE system was developed and succeeded the SMART program, differentiating itself by legally requiring participation by all physicians and patients using isotretinoin.

Generally, when a physician and his or her patient decide to pursue treatment with isotretinoin, they are required to sign paperwork to register with the iPLEDGE system. People are classified as "patients who can get pregnant" and "patients who cannot get pregnant" within the iPLEDGE system when registering. This classification is important because each group has different specific requirements while using the iPLEDGE system.

For those who can get pregnant, iPLEDGE requires that they pick two birth control methods, which can include abstinence, condom use, oral contraceptives, and implantable devices, among others. In addition, two doctor-administered pregnancy tests are required over the course of two consecutive months to minimize the risk of unknown or unexpected pregnancy before starting the medication. Following the two negative pregnancy tests, users are required to take an online comprehension test to show that they understand the requirements of the iPLEDGE system prior to taking isotretinoin. It is only after completing all of these requirements that people are able to be authorized to pick up and use isotretinoin. Finally, after every month of using the medication, another pregnancy test must be done under the supervision of a doctor to prove that pregnancy has not occurred while using isotretinoin.

On the other hand, people who are classified as patients who cannot get pregnant still must see their physician on a monthly basis under the iPLEDGE program, but they are not required to take any pregnancy tests or pass a comprehension exam.

While the goal of minimizing birth defects and preventing negative outcomes while using isotretinoin is a very important and reasonable objective, the iPLEDGE system has also received a significant amount of criticism for a number of reasons. Many people point out that the iPLEDGE system imposes a number of requirements that can make getting access to isotretinoin very difficult, especially for people with less financial resources and support. In fact, it has been objectively shown that iPLEDGE significantly increases the cost of health care for people who require isotretinoin therapy due to the increased number of doctor visits, pregnancy tests, and administrative burden. For people who are not able to afford these additional costs, getting access to isotretinoin can be extremely difficult or even impossible in the United States.

Another very common criticism of the iPLEDGE program is that it is inherently sexist because the vast majority of the additional requirements imposed by the program fall upon the group identified as patients who can get pregnant. Most females with acne fall within this category and are therefore required to go through significantly more steps to get access to isotretinoin. Because of this, it has been pointed out that these additional steps can serve as a barrier that prevents females and other people who can get pregnant from getting access to a medication that they would significantly benefit from.

Despite these criticisms of iPLEDGE, the overall rate of pregnancy for people using isotretinoin has been minimal in the modern era. For example, the most recent study of the iPLEDGE system showed that less than a fraction of a percent of people get pregnant while on the iPLEDGE system and using isotretinoin. Although the ultimate goal is to have zero pregnancies and no negative outcomes, the iPLEDGE system is a tool that is meant to prevent harm to all people who use isotretinoin.

40. How is hormonal acne treated differently than other types of acne?

There is significant overlap between the treatment of hormonal acne and treatment of the other commonly seen forms of acne. However, there are some differences that are important to be aware of.

Although all forms of acne are influenced by the balance of hormones in the body, especially the levels of testosterone and the other androgens, hormonal acne is especially influenced by these levels. Therefore, controlling the level of hormones in the body and correcting any imbalances is an important aspect of the treatment of hormonal acne. In addition, hormonal acne is unique from the more classic forms of acne in that it tends to be resistant to classic treatment regimens while responding very well to treatment regimens that add on hormone-influencing medications.

Hormonal acne is still primarily treated with the use of medications commonly used in the treatment of classic acne. Topical benzoyl peroxide, topical retinoid products, and appropriate skin hygiene are important cornerstones for the treatment of both regular acne and hormonal acne. However, hormonal acne also requires treatment with medications that block or otherwise impact the excess activity of androgen hormones, especially testosterone and dihydrotestosterone (DHT).

One of the most common medications that is used to regulate hormone levels in the body for people who suffer from hormonal acne is oral contraceptives. The regular use of oral contraceptives allows the body's cycle of hormone levels to become more balanced and normalized, helping to reduce hormonal acne. In addition, the pregnancy-prevention aspect of oral contraceptives allows females with hormonal acne to protect themselves against unexpected pregnancy while also treating their acne. Importantly, however, oral contraceptives can influence other aspects of the body in profound ways, and some women are unable to tolerate side effects such as tiredness, nausea, weight changes, and breast soreness. Thankfully, there are other options for treating hormonal acne.

Another one of the most commonly used medications in treating hormonal acne—in addition to the staple medications like benzoyl peroxide and retinoids—is spironolactone. Interestingly, spironolactone was first developed as a medication for controlling blood pressure by influencing the function of a specific portion of the kidneys. However, it was later observed that spironolactone also had a potent role in blocking the production of androgen hormones in the body, helping to regulate hormone levels in people who had excess levels of testosterone, DHT, and other androgens in their body. It is this anti-androgen effect of spironolactone that makes it tremendously useful in women who suffer from hormonal acne.

In addition to hormonal acne, spironolactone has been used to treat other conditions influenced by excess levels of testosterone and DHT, such as excess facial hair or certain patterns of hair loss. Importantly, the ability of spironolactone to reduce the activity of androgens in the body means that it is not safe to use during pregnancy due to the risk of birth defects. It is also not commonly used for the treatment acne in men because it can result in enlargement of the normal breast tissue (gynecomastia) and loss of sex drive as well as changes in the normal balance of the body's electrolyte levels.

One of the biggest challenges facing people with hormonal acne is that the condition can be very resistant to treatment when antihormonal medicines are not used. In fact, one of the signs that a person is suffering from hormonal acne is that his or her acne is not getting better despite treatment with benzoyl peroxide and retinoids. In addition, women who report cycling of their acne flares in parallel with their menstrual cycle and complain of acne that lines their chin and jaw are more likely to have the hormonal form of acne that requires treatment with hormone-influencing medications to be effectively treated.

Thankfully, once a diagnosis of hormonal acne is made and treatment with oral contraceptive pills or spironolactone is initiated, improvement in the acne and the skin can be seen rather quickly. For women who add oral contraceptives to their regimen, improvement in acne can be seen within a few months. For those who decide to use spironolactone, acne and skin oiliness can improve as quickly as a few weeks. Ultimately, the majority of women with hormonal acne see an improvement in their acne with these medications. One study showed that approximately a third of people on these medications show clearing of their acne, and another third experience significant improvement, with only about one in ten people not seeing any improvement. Therefore, hormonally active medications such as oral contraceptives and spironolactone are essential parts of an effective treatment regimen for people with hormonal acne.

41. Can light therapy be helpful in treating acne?

Lasers and light therapy are becoming an increasingly popular method for treating acne in the modern era. Although medications remain the most commonly prescribed treatments for acne, the appeal of lasers and light therapy in minimizing side effects and reducing the number of steps in daily skin-care routines has attracted many people with acne.

A wide variety of laser and light therapy machines have been developed over the past few decades. In fact, there are thousands of such devices available for purchase by consumers as well as medical offices and hospitals. Generally, the laser and light therapy devices available to physicians' offices and hospitals are much stronger and more effective than those available for purchase and use at home.

The most popular machines available for at-home use are blue, red, and combined light devices. These are able to be purchased for use at home, which makes them a convenient and more affordable option for people who want to be able to treat their acne in the comfort of their own home. However, the visible form of light used by these machines is rather weak and is not effective against most forms of acne. In fact, neither blackheads, whiteheads, acne cysts, nor nodules are treated by this visible form of light. Although classic pimples can respond well to light therapy, effective use often takes up to an hour of treatment multiple times a day for several weeks. This makes it an impractical option for many people who do not have that amount of free time in their daily routine.

On the other hand, there are a wide range of highly effective devices that are able to be used by physicians' offices and hospitals. One of the most common categories of laser and light therapy devices is called photodynamic therapy (PDT). In PDT, a solution is applied to acne-prone skin for several minutes to hours to make that area of skin more sensitive to light therapy. Then, a dermatologist uses the laser or light device to treat the skin with a powerful and focused amount of energy.

Photodynamic therapy has been shown to be rather effective for most forms of acne. In fact, it can be especially beneficial for people who have acne that has been resistant to topical and oral medications. For this group of people, having an additional option for treating their acne can be a life-changing thing. Unfortunately, however, the cost of receiving the treatment and the requirement for multiple treatments to see an improvement in acne can make PDT an unrealistic option for many people.

Although the cost of PDT can vary significantly based on the location, one session can cost anywhere from $100 to over $400, and effective treatment of acne can take multiple sessions. Since PDT is seen as a cosmetic procedure by most insurance companies, people who pursue treatment are required to pay for the treatment on their own. In addition, the skin becomes very sensitive after treatment, so direct sunlight must be avoided for up to forty-eight hours following treatment. During this time, the skin can be uncomfortable and painful as well. Therefore, while PDT can be an incredibly effective option, especially for people who have exhausted other treatment choices, it does come with significant barriers and drawbacks.

In addition to treating acne with light and laser therapies, there are a variety of laser machines that are incredibly effective for treating acne scars and other long-term changes in the skin associated with acne. Even after people stop having acne, their scars and other skin changes can cause them to experience significant distress and embarrassment. Therefore, having an option for treating their scarring is very important.

Some of the laser therapies used to treat acne scarring include fractionated resurfacing lasers, which help to induce collagen formation and normalize the skin surface, as well as pulsed dye lasers, which cause blood vessels to constrict, reducing the redness of skin and scars. Although these treatments share the same concerns regarding cost, discomfort, and the need for multiple sessions, they can be incredibly effective for people who are troubled by significant scarring after their acne has improved.

42. What cosmetic treatments can help with acne?

For most people, acne responds well to treatment with topical and oral medications. However, there are some people who are not able to find significant improvement in their skin despite trying different medication regimens and getting help from a trained dermatologist. In these situations, there are a variety of cosmetic treatments that can help improve the appearance of the skin and keep acne under control. In fact, there is a whole specialty in dermatology, known as cosmetic dermatology, that is focused on cosmetic options for the treatment and management of skin issues.

In addition to the laser and light therapies available for the treatment of acne, there are a plethora of other options available in the cosmetic world of dermatology. Skin resurfacing is one popular option, which involves removal of the top layer of the skin to even out texture and stimulate new growth of collagen and other components of healthy skin. Although skin resurfacing can be done with the use of specialized laser devices, chemical peels, dermabrasion, and even microdermabrasion are options available to people who are interested in the cosmetic procedure.

In chemical peels, special chemical solutions are applied to the face and other affected areas to irritate and cause the top layer of the skin to pull apart from the surrounding skin. This helps to exfoliate the skin, dissolve built-up skin oils, and unclog blocked pores. Chemical peels often take less than an hour and allow people to even their skin texture over the course of multiple treatments. The most commonly used chemicals for these types of peels include salicylic acid and glycolic acid.

On the other hand, dermabrasion and microdermabrasion involve the use of a tool that is dragged across the skin surface to remove the top layer of skin. The primary difference between dermabrasion and microdermabrasion is that dermabrasion goes slightly deeper into the skin. However, both dermabrasion and microdermabrasion help to even the skin texture, stimulate new skin growth, and improve whiteheads, blackheads, and other acne bumps. The procedure can be uncomfortable, so many dermatologists use numbing gels and creams to help minimize the discomfort. Interestingly, dermabrasion and microdermabrasion are also effective for treating acne scars, and an improvement in acne and scarring can be seen within several weeks.

Another effective option for people with acne who have nodules and cysts that are not responding effectively to medications is injections. Steroid injections can be incredibly effective at helping to reduce the discomfort associated with acne cysts, and they can help cysts and nodules resolve on their own over the course of several days and weeks. After steroid injections, acne bumps soften and flatten, and pain can significantly decrease. Although steroid injections can be incredibly helpful for people with nodulocystic acne, steroid medications can cause thinning of the skin, and the skin color may become uneven or splotchy. Therefore, steroid injections should not be the first choice of treatment but rather an option after other choices have been exhausted or when there is significant discomfort and pain.

Although cosmetic treatments for acne and acne scars can be incredibly effective, they are not often covered by health insurance companies, which means that pursuing treatment from a cosmetic dermatologist can be expensive and challenging. In addition, most forms of cosmetic treatments for acne do not prevent acne from happening in the first place but, rather, are focused on helping the acne look better once it has happened. Therefore, people who pursue treatment from a cosmetic dermatologist for their acne should continue to treat and manage their acne with the use of topical and oral acne medications. This can help to prevent the onset of new acne bumps while getting treatment for current and old acne lesions.

43. Does alternative medicine offer any effective treatments for acne?

There is a lighthearted joke that many health-care professionals know that goes, "What do you call alternative medicine that works?" The answer, jokingly, is "Medicine!" One of the reasons that this joke is popular is because many treatments sold under the label of alternative medicine have not been shown to be effective and sometimes have even been found to be harmful. Therefore, the medical community has slowly moved away from recommending alternative medicines, instead preferring to focus on complementary therapies. Whereas alternative medicine means that the person has chosen a nontraditional option instead of the classic recommendation, complementary therapy means that the person can use both the classic option and the alternative option together under the supervision of a health-care professional.

Complementary therapy is preferred because the classic treatments for acne, such as benzoyl peroxide, topical and oral retinoids, and hormonal medications, have been shown to be the most effective and safest treatments available. Therefore, complementary therapies should be used in addition to the classic treatments to maximize the chance for success in treating acne.

As the treatment of acne has evolved over the past few decades, the number of complementary treatment options has also increased significantly. Many people report significant improvement of their acne with the use of these complementary therapies, but there have been few scientific studies that prove their effectiveness. However, many people, dermatologists, and other skin-care professionals recommend a variety of complementary products as part of a daily skin-care routine.

Tea tree oil is a very popular complementary therapy used by people who suffer from acne. Tea tree oil is an essential oil from the leaves of a specific tree that is native to Australia, and it has long been thought that it can help with acne. One study that compared the effectiveness of using tea tree oil to benzoyl peroxide found that people in both groups experienced improvement of their acne over a long period of time, but the tea tree oil caused a little less irritation in the skin. However, tea tree oil can cause significant skin irritation or even an allergic reaction in select people, so careful use is recommended. In fact, many complementary therapies involve the use of essential oils, which can all trigger allergic or irritant reactions in sensitive skin; therefore, caution with most complementary therapies is recommended.

Certain forms of honey have also been explored as a complementary therapy for the treatment of acne. Most types of raw honey have been shown to function as natural antimicrobials that help to kill bacteria. This is because honey has a chemical called glucuronic acid that eventually converts to hydrogen peroxide on the surface of the skin, which can help to kill bacteria. Although the research around the use of honey for the treatment of acne is sparse, some people report that it helps to soothe their skin and makes them feel better. However, it is important to use raw honey when attempting to use honey for the treatment of acne because processing honey can greatly reduce its antimicrobial effectiveness and render it ineffective.

Some people also appreciate the contribution of older and more traditional medical systems when treating their acne. For example, Ayurvedic medicine is one popular traditional system of medicine that has its roots in the Indian subcontinent. In Ayurvedic medicine, the cause of acne is attributed to an imbalance in the elemental energies of the body, specifically too much of the fire energy in the body. Therefore, Ayurvedic practitioners recommend soothing the body's fire energy through the use of increased water intake, regular facial washing, and yoga and other forms of sweating exercises.

Acupuncture is another form of complementary therapy that has its roots in traditional Chinese medicine. Acupuncture involves the use of thin needles that are inserted into the body to influence and improve health. Although many research studies have shown that acupuncture is a pseudoscience and is not effective for the treatment of most conditions, some people report positive personal experiences with it. It is postulated that acupuncture can help to influence hormone levels in the body and help to improve acne through this way. Unfortunately, this has not been shown to be the case in most research studies evaluating the topic.

There are also a wide variety of other complementary therapies that have been recommended for the treatment of acne, including wet cupping and the use of bee venom and chemicals such as brewer's yeast and fruit tannins. There has been conflicting evidence regarding the use of these techniques, but some people report feeling a benefit from their use. In these situations, people are often recommended to continue what works for them, unless they start to experience negative side effects.

44. What are the common side effects of acne treatment?

The treatments available for acne are generally safe with only mild side effects. However, no medical therapy is perfect, and these side effects can definitely impact people's lives. Therefore, it is important to be aware of the different side effects that can accompany the use of the various medical treatments available for acne.

Benzoyl peroxide is one of the most commonly prescribed acne medications in the world. Although it is incredibly effective in managing acne, especially when combined with other acne medications, it does carry a number of different side effects. The most common negative effect of benzoyl peroxide is that it mildly dries the skin and can cause some skin sensitivity. This effect is worst when first starting the medicine, so most dermatologists recommend starting once a day for a week before building up to twice a day use. Although much rarer, some people do develop an allergic reaction to benzoyl peroxide, and use of this medicine should be stopped in those situations.

Another commonly used class of medications in the treatment of acne is topical retinoids. This group can cause similar dryness and irritation as benzoyl peroxide, but it can be more significant. Some people also experience skin tingling, warmth, or burning immediately after applying topical retinoids to their skin. Similar to benzoyl peroxide, these side effects are worst during the first few weeks of starting the medication, and most dermatologists recommend slowly and carefully building up to regular use.

In addition, topical retinoids change the way that the skin reacts to light, which can cause skin to become extremely sensitive to sun exposure. Therefore, people can develop severe sunburns if they use retinoids during the day or without adequate sunscreen. To reduce the risk of this happening, people are encouraged to use retinoid medications as part of their evening routine after the sun has set and to wear sunscreen whenever they are exposed to sunlight.

Although topical and oral retinoids share similar side effect profiles, oral retinoids tend to exhibit those side effects to a greater degree. In addition, oral retinoids can cause significant flaring of acne over the whole body when first starting the medication. Oral retinoids have also been shown to cause birth defects when they are used during pregnancy. To minimize the risk of getting pregnant while taking oral retinoids, the U.S. government has developed the iPLEDGE system, which requires the use of birth control and frequent pregnancy tests while taking oral retinoids, particularly isotretinoin (Accutane).

Unfortunately, most people experience some of these side effects while treating their acne with medications. In the majority of cases, these side effects are limited to mild skin dryness and some flaring of their acne while first starting medication therapy. Thankfully, most people experience improvement in these symptoms after their body adjusts to the medication regimen, and they begin to experience less dryness and irritation as their acne subsides and improves. Therefore, people who start treatment with acne medications should not feel disheartened or hopeless if they do not see immediate improvement in the days to weeks after starting therapy. Most people will see a significant improvement in their acne, but they will need to wait several weeks for it to become apparent that their skin condition is improving.

45. How long does it typically take to effectively treat acne?

Acne often happens on the most visible and important parts of the body, such as the face, neck, and shoulders. This can make it very frustrating for people who are distressed by their acne and feel embarrassment and shame at the change in their appearance. Therefore, it can be very hard to be patient and give acne medication regimens time to work effectively to improve and resolve acne. However, almost all of the effective treatments for acne do not work immediately; they require time to improve skin from the inside out.

For people with mild to moderate acne who begin treatment of their acne with a topical regimen, it can take up to four to six weeks to begin to see their acne clear. This is because the skin takes significant time to change its behavior and begin to normalize in response to medications. It can be frustrating for people who bear through the side effects of skin dryness and acne flaring to not see an improvement in their acne for weeks and weeks, but this is a normal part of treating acne. People should be counseled regarding expectations by their dermatologist.

For people with more severe forms of acne that require treatment with oral isotretinoin, the time frame for clearing of acne can be even longer. Most people who start isotretinoin will see a significant worsening of their acne over the first few weeks, with their acne bumps becoming more red, inflamed, and uncomfortable. However, most people begin to see their acne clear significantly within approximately three months. In fact, eight to twelve weeks is considered the peak effect time for isotretinoin therapy.

Importantly, a minority of people require up to four or five months of treatment to see the full effect of isotretinoin therapy on their skin. Thankfully, isotretinoin therapy requires close supervision by a physician who can help to guide and determine how long the therapy should be continued. Some people may experience flaring of their acne once they stop treatment with isotretinoin, but an additional shorter course of treatment with isotretinoin can help to resolve this.

For the scarring left by acne once it heals, especially in people with moderate to severe forms of acne, the amount of time it takes to improve can vary significantly based on the specific treatment used. For people who use dermabrasion and microdermabrasion, the skin begins to heal and recover over the course of a couple of weeks, and the appearance of the scars can continue to improve until approximately six to eight weeks following treatment. For those who use laser and light therapies, several treatments over the course of weeks and months are required before seeing a significant improvement. Chemical peels are similar in that they require multiple treatments over a long period of time to see progressive improvements in skin texture and healing.

Although seeing an improvement in acne and acne scarring takes time, and ample amounts of patience are recommended for all people who pursue treatment of their acne, some signs that acne is not responding appropriately to treatment include no improvement in acne after several months of treatment, new worsening of acne after the initial starting period of treatment, and changes in the acne that could be concerning for an infection or a new skin condition. In each of these situations, a dermatologist or other physician should be consulted to review the treatment and make recommendations regarding the next steps. In some cases, changing the treatment may be required, and some people require additional medications to get control of their acne.

46. Is treating acne expensive?

Health care in the United States is a complex and confusing system that involves health insurance companies, health-care providers, copays, deductibles, and many other complicated features. Therefore, treating acne can range from being very affordable to very expensive, depending on the specific circumstances and insurance coverage that is available. In addition, the particular treatments required and the severity of the acne can significantly impact how affordable or expensive it is.

For the most common forms of acne, treatment does not need to be expensive. Most benzoyl peroxide washes are available over the counter, which means that a doctor's visit or formal prescription is not required. In addition, many companies offer generic forms of medications, such as benzoyl peroxide, which are cheaper than the same brand name products. For example, Target carries a generic benzoyl peroxide wash that is only a few dollars for a month's supply.

Alongside benzoyl peroxide, retinoids are the most commonly used medications for treating acne, and, thankfully, adapalene, also known as Differin, was recently approved for over-the-counter use, making it one of the most powerful retinoids that can be used without requiring a doctor's visit or prescription. Therefore, most people with acne who have mild to moderate acne can self-treat their condition with over-the-counter medications such as benzoyl peroxide and adapalene for approximately $10 to $15 a month, which is affordable for a significant percentage of the population.

Also, most people have some form of insurance coverage, whether through school, work, family, or the regulated health-care marketplace, which means that seeing a general physician or dermatologist to help coordinate the treatment of their acne is either partially or fully covered by insurance. Many people are required to make a copay before seeing their physician, while others are able to visit physicians at no cost. The best way to estimate the cost of a physician's visit is to read the insurance paperwork that states the different costs associated with an insurance plan.

Regardless of how affordable treating common acne might be for the average person, the cost can rise significantly when acne is more severe and requires more aggressive treatment. For example, someone with severe acne can require treatment with isotretinoin, which requires monthly visits with a dermatologist, monthly blood work, and monthly pregnancy tests for those who are able to become pregnant. This means that a treatment with isotretinoin over the course of six months could cost upward of a thousand dollars with insurance and thousands of dollars if covering the cost of medicine, doctor's visits, and blood work out of pocket. In almost all cases, the cosmetic treatments for acne scarring after acne goes away are not covered by insurance, and these can often cost hundreds of dollars, if not thousands of dollars.

Therefore, the cost of adequately treating and improving acne is extremely dependent on the severity of the acne and the particular circumstances surrounding each individual, including their specific insurance coverage, the medicines that they need, and the amount of follow-up that they require. Thankfully, for the majority of people with mild to moderate acne, treatment is fairly affordable and attainable. Even for people with severe acne, a combination of adequate insurance coverage and in-network health care can help to make treatment of acne more affordable. However, the structure of the health-care system and the way that health care is paid for in the United States continues to remain a complicated and challenging topic.

Managing the Skin after Acne

47. Can acne reoccur?

For the majority of people with acne, especially adolescents and young adults, acne is a skin condition that comes and goes in waves. Although treatment with acne medications can significantly improve existing acne and reduce the amount and severity of acne flares, most people will continue to experience periodic acne bumps and pimples that need additional treatment. Therefore, acne is not typically thought of as a condition that is *cured* but rather one that is better *controlled* with the use of medications and other treatments. However, most people will experience a significant reduction in the number of acne flares that they experience once they transition out of adolescence and enter true adulthood, as hormone levels in the body balance out and the body's oil-producing sebaceous glands normalize their behavior.

People who use topical or oral medications to manage their acne can experience flares of their acne after stopping the use of acne treatments. Oftentimes, people start using benzoyl peroxide and a retinoid serum for several weeks to months until their acne significantly improves, then they decide to stop using the products because their acne is better. In these situations, acne can return and cause significant distress and frustration. Therefore, it is important to continue to use an effective acne regimen even after the acne clears so that the skin can continue to be under the

influence of normalizing medications that help prevent acne from forming in the first place.

Another common period of recurrence is following treatment with
isotretinoin (Accutane), the oral medication used to manage severe
forms of acne as well as acne that has not responded to other medicines.
Isotretinoin involves a very intense course of treatment with a powerful
medicine that requires regular doctor's visits, blood work, and pregnancy
tests for those who are able to become pregnant. Therefore, it can be
extremely frustrating for people to complete several months of treatment
with isotretinoin with significant improvement of their acne and then to
experience a bad acne flare once they finish their treatment.

Recently, new research has indicated that a longer treatment length
with higher doses of isotretinoin can help to prevent the recurrence of
acne following a treatment course. In fact, about half of people following
the old dosing guidelines for isotretinoin experienced a relapse of their
acne. Although only a very small portion of people required restarting
the medication, this was still a frustrating and disheartening experience.
However, the new longer length and higher dose treatment course has
been shown to reduce the rate of recurrence from approximately half
to only a quarter of people. This advance in the understanding of how
to best use isotretinoin means that more people are satisfied with their
results following treatment with the medication.

Another important factor that contributes to recurrences of acne is the
presence of individual-specific acne triggers. Most people are able to identify some particular triggers that tend to incite acne flares in their skin.
For some people, sleeping facedown, having longer hair, eating unhealthy
foods, or missing their face washing routine are the most common triggers
that worsen their acne. For others, excessive sweating during sports or
exercise, sharing makeup products with others, or specific types of weather,
such as humid or hot summer afternoons, are the most common contributors to their acne flares. Whatever the specific situation, it is important to
take steps to avoid being exposed to those triggers because they can cause
acne to flare even while it is being treated with medications.

48. Does acne have any long-term impact on the skin?

The skin is one of the most dynamic and alive organs of the body. It has
to be so to respond to the needs of protecting the rest of the body and
keeping the outside environment from disrupting the balance within the
body. Unlike the brain, where many of the brain's cells can last for several

years up to an entire lifetime, the vast majority of the cells on the surface of the skin live a measly three weeks before being completely replaced by new skin cells.

Thankfully, this rapid and short-lived life span for skin cells means that acne does not negatively affect the skin over the long term, as long as it is limited to the surface of the skin. For people with mild to moderate acne who are able to effectively treat their acne early with the use of medications, their skin does not experience any long-term negative effects once the acne resolves. Although some people, especially those with darker skin tones, can experience discoloration of their skin for several months in spots where they experienced acne, this discoloration is temporary and, ultimately, completely resolves.

However, the most important long-term impact that acne can have on the skin is when it affects deeper portions of the skin, underneath the surface. The cells that are responsible for organizing the structure of the skin and producing the new cells that form the surface of the skin live within these deeper portions. It is only when acne disrupts these cells and causes them to be destroyed or to change their function that acne can cause significant long-term effects on the skin.

The most common circumstances where acne affects the deeper portions of the skin involves moderate to severe forms of acne or nodulocystic acne, where the inflammation and skin damage is so severe that it extends into the deeper parts of the skin. In these situations, the inflammation causes changes in the structure of the connective tissue that organizes and supports the overlying skin. This contributes to the bumpy and uneven texture of acne scars in the skin of people who suffered from severe acne.

Unfortunately, when people develop this type of acne scarring, the changes in the skin are permanent and do not resolve without treatment. This is because the new skin cells that are being formed are organized into uneven layers by the deeper, damaged portions of skin. While acne itself can be frustrating and challenging to deal with, people can experience similar levels of distress, frustration, embarrassment, and anguish when dealing with the long-term consequences of acne scarring.

Thankfully, there are treatments available that can help with improving the appearance of acne scars. Specifically, many cosmetic treatments are available that target the uneven texture of acne scars and help to make the skin more even and uniform. For example, one form of acne scar treatment is subcision, which involves the use of needles targeted underneath the acne scars. Injuring the area underneath the acne scars can temporarily help to promote collagen formation and encourage new repairs of the tissue underneath the depressed areas of scarring, which serves to elevate the depressed skin, allowing it to be more even with the surrounding skin.

49. Why can skin become lighter or darker after acne goes away?

The inflammation caused by acne can profoundly affect the color of the skin, even after the original acne bumps have improved and gone away. This is because the inflammation seen in acne affects melanocytes, the cells responsible for creating and spreading the pigment that gives skin its color.

Melanocytes are responsible for the production of melanin, which gives color to the skin, eyes, and hair. Once melanin is produced, it is transported to nearby keratinocytes, which are the cells that make up the top layer of the skin. This distribution of pigment helps to protect the cells of the skin against sunlight, which is a powerful form of ultraviolet (UV) radiation that can cause cell damage.

Unfortunately, however, melanocytes are very sensitive to a variety of factors, including significant temperature changes, inflammation, hormones, and even age. When acne causes inflammation in the skin, it can cause melanocytes to change their production of pigment, which leads to the abnormal dark or light spots that are associated with acne. This is especially common among people with darker skin tones, where such color changes are more obvious and visible. This phenomenon most often causes darkening of the skin around the area where acne bumps used to be and is termed *postinflammatory hyperpigmentation*, which means darkening of the skin following inflammation.

In postinflammatory hyperpigmentation, inflammation in the skin because of acne causes melanocytes to increase their production of melanin pigment as well as increase the amount of pigment that is transferred to surrounding keratinocytes. Although the exact mechanism that causes melanocytes to increase the production and transportation of pigments because of inflammation is not clear, it has been shown that many of the chemicals involved in inflammation also affect melanocytes. Cytokines, chemokines, and other chemicals are responsible for controlling inflammation in the body, and they have been shown to also affect melanocyte function. Subsequently, the increased production and transportation of melanin by melanocytes affected by inflammation contributes to the development of skin darkening in areas where acne bumps were.

Conversely, inflammation and damage to the skin can also cause the opposite phenomenon, *postinflammatory hypopigmentation*, where inflammation causes abnormal lightening of the skin. The reason why some people's melanocytes respond to inflammation by increasing pigment production and other people's melanocytes respond by decreasing pigment production is unclear. However, it has been theorized that there are genetic factors responsible for predicting how a person's melanocytes will react to inflammation. It has been shown, though, that damage to the skin that is severe enough to kill melanocytes, rather than injure them, will always result in hypopigmentation or skin lightening rather than skin darkening.

Although the pigment changes that occur as a result of inflammation caused by acne can be troublesome and distressing for many people, the good news is that the changes are temporary. Eventually, the behavior of melanocytes after inflammation returns to normal, and the skin regains an even coloration. However, it is important to appreciate that the process of returning to normal function takes several months, and people can experience postinflammatory skin color changes for long periods of time before their skin color normalizes.

There are options for people who suffer from postinflammatory hyperpigmentation and do not want to wait several months for their skin tone to return to normal. There are a variety of lightening treatments that can be effective, including medications such as hydroquinone, azelaic acid, and even tretinoin. In addition, chemical peels, laser treatments, and light therapies have been shown to help with hyperpigmentation as well, but it is important to ensure that they do not cause additional damage to melanocytes and worsen the problem.

Another important step for people with postinflammatory hyperpigmentation is avoiding sun exposure and tanning. Exposure to sunlight causes additional darkening of the skin and can exacerbate dark spots and make uneven skin tone even more visible and problematic. Therefore, the regular use of sunscreen products and avoidance of sunlight during peak hours of the day are an important part of managing postinflammatory hyperpigmentation.

50. What causes acne scarring?

One of the most serious acne complications is acne scarring. The scarring that is left after acne goes away is permanent, if left untreated, and can be highly distressing to individuals.

Although not everyone who has acne will develop scarring from it, there are a few risk factors that increase the chance of experiencing scarring. The risk of developing scarring from acne significantly increases based on how inflammatory the acne is. When there are lots of cysts, nodules, and areas of inflammation that penetrate deep into the skin, the chances of scarring are much higher. Thankfully, as long as inflammatory acne is treated early and effectively, scarring can be minimized. However, delays in treatment increase the risk of scarring. The longer that a person has inflammatory acne, the greater their chance of scarring.

In addition, picking, squeezing, or popping acne pimples and cysts is a very dangerous habit that significantly increases the chance of acne scarring the skin. This is because those behaviors increase the amount of inflammation in the area as well as directly damage the deeper portions of the skin. Also, having a direct relative who developed acne scars is a risk factor for scarring, as genetics play a large role in determining who experiences scarring and who does not.

To understand the reason that some people develop scarring from their acne, it is necessary to understand the structure and function of the skin. The top layer of the skin is supported by a framework of connective tissue deeper down. This deeper layer helps to maintain and organize the layers that are higher up. One of the most important materials in the deeper layers of the skin is collagen, which gives the skin support and substance. When acne breakouts penetrate into the skin and the underlying supportive layers, it can cause significant damage to the collagen and other connective tissue. As the body attempts to heal this damage, it produces collagen and a variety of other substances to replace the damaged areas. However, if the amount of collagen and other factors are not the same as they used to be, this can contribute to scarring and visible differences in the scar as compared to the surrounding skin.

For example, people with acne scars that are depressed, or lower than the surrounding skin, suffer from too little collagen in the areas of their scarring. In these circumstances, the body was unable to create the correct amount of collagen, and the scarred area is not supported well enough to be level with the surrounding skin. This can create an visible uneven texture in the skin that is undesirable to many people.

On the other hand, in some people, the healing response to acne damage causes too much collagen to be created, leading to a raised acne scar. As the underlying supportive tissue is packed with too much collagen, it causes the overlying area to bulge out from the surrounding skin. Although this form of acne scarring can affect anyone, it is more common in people who have skin of color, including Africans, African Americans, Hispanics, and Asians.

While it is impossible to always prevent acne from scarring, the most important steps that can be taken include treating acne early and effectively as well as avoiding picking at acne bumps. When concerned about acne scarring, speaking with a dermatologist early on is always an appropriate next step.

51. How common are acne scars?

Although most people who experience acne do not ever go on to have scarring, the development of acne scars is a common and unfortunate reality for many people. It is especially troubling for people who have severe inflammatory acne and develop extensive scarring that is difficult to cover with makeup and highly visible. While acne is not a lifelong condition for most people, acne scars are unfortunately permanent if left untreated and can be a large contributor to unhappiness and worsened mental health.

While the vast majority of people will experience acne at some point in their life, approximately one out of every five people with acne will develop acne scarring. Some recent studies have suggested that the rate of acne scarring might even be meaningfully higher than this. This means that a significant portion of the population develops and lives with acne scarring, which is a permanent change in the skin, unlike acne, which can come and go.

In addition, the rate of acne scarring can be much higher when considering people who have the more severe form of acne. For example, people with moderate or severe acne develop acne scarring at an increased rate of almost 30%. This means that nearly one in every three people with moderate to severe acne will develop permanent scarring from their acne. For people who have even more severe forms of acne, such as acne fulminans or nodulocystic acne, the rate of acne scarring can be even higher than this. In fact, people with severe nodulocystic acne are almost always left with significant areas of scarring on their cheeks and face because the inflammation always extends deep into the skin, where it can affect collagen and connective tissue, leaving scarring behind.

Although the rates of acne in the general population have been increasing over the past few decades, especially among nonadolescents, the development of newer treatments and approaches to minimize acne scarring have helped to control the rise of long-term scarring. The past few decades have led to a significant expansion in the availability and affordability of medical and cosmetic treatments for acne scarring, including laser therapies, light devices, resurfacing treatments, and dermabrasion techniques. Studies that have examined the effectiveness of these treatments have found that a majority of people who seek treatment for their acne scarring are able to see moderate to significant improvement of their scars. Therefore, acne scarring has become less of a permanent, life-changing phenomenon and more of a curable medical condition that can be resolved with the appropriate treatment.

52. Is there a way to minimize the chance of developing acne scars?

There are a few important ways to minimize the chance of developing acne scars. While effective treatments for improving acne scars have been developed over the past few decades, the best approach to acne scarring remains prevention rather than treatment. By preventing the development of scarring, the need for additional medical care and cosmetic treatments can be minimized and the quality of the skin can be maintained. As Benjamin Franklin famously advised, an ounce of prevention is worth a pound of cure.

In regard to the best ways to minimize the chances of developing acne scars, two important steps stand out as essential. The first key step to avoiding acne scarring is to get effective medical treatment for acne early on. Waiting for acne to worsen and become highly inflamed before getting treatment means that the skin is exposed to significant amounts of damaging inflammation. This increases the risk of developing scarring, even if effective treatment for the acne is eventually received later on. By intervening early and preventing inflammation from developing and worsening, the risk of acne scarring is significantly reduced. As part of this approach, continuing to use a maintenance treatment regimen of medications such as benzoyl peroxide and a retinoid cream, even when the skin is healthy, can help to prevent a recurrence of acne and reduce the chances of scarring.

The second important step for reducing the chances of developing scarring from acne is sometimes one of the hardest things to do for people who get significant pimples and zits. Not picking and scratching at acne bumps is one of the most crucial parts of avoiding acne scarring, and it is one of the most challenging things to do, especially because inflamed skin sends lots of itch and discomfort signals to the brain. These signals

make us crave picking at acne bumps. However, by scratching and picking at pimples and zits, there is a lot of extra damage caused to the skin,
and the amount of inflammation in acne significantly increases. In fact,
this can multiply the amount of scarring that happens because of acne
by extending the damage and inflammation deeper into the skin than it
would have ever reached on its own. Therefore, avoiding touching and
disturbing acne bumps is an essential step for anyone hoping to reduce
their chances of scarring from acne.

Some practical steps to help make pimples and zits more bearable
and to avoid scratching include using warm water for washing the face
and using anti-itch lotions and creams, such as aloe vera and calamine.
However, it can sometimes be impossible to 100% avoid picking at acne
bumps, especially when such behaviors have become a habit. Therefore,
in moments when people become aware of their picking, changing activities and finding another way to occupy the hands and the mind can be
very helpful. This constant correction also helps to train the brain not to
pick at acne bumps mindlessly. In fact, for some people who have a very
challenging time changing their picking behaviors, getting health from a
therapist who practices cognitive behavioral therapy (CBT) can be tremendously helpful. CBT uses the same process of correcting thoughts and
actions whenever we become aware of them to effect change for the better, and this form of therapy has been successfully used in the treatment of
excess acne-picking behaviors.

Despite getting early treatment for acne and avoiding picking at acne
bumps, some people may still develop acne scars. In fact, genetic predis-
position is thought to play a large role in determining who develops acne
scars and who does not. Some people are thought to be more prone to
developing scarring from their acne, and people who have close family
members with acne scars are at the greatest risk. Therefore, while it is
impossible to entirely reduce the risk of developing acne scarring, it is still
important to take the steps that are within our control to minimize the
chances of scarring.

If acne scarring does occur, getting treatment early on, soon after the
acne has subsided, can help to get the best treatment results. As time
goes on, scars can become more fixed and difficult to treat. The collagen
and connective tissue become more engrained and interconnected with
the surrounding skin. By getting treatment for acne scars early on, the
number of treatments required and the chances of successfully improving
the appearance of the skin are optimized. As with all things related to
the skin, speaking with a dermatologist and seeking professional advice is
never the wrong decision.

53. Are acne scars permanent?

While acne itself is not permanent, and most people tend to experience an improvement of their acne as they grow older and leave adolescence and early adulthood, acne scarring is usually permanent if it is not treated. This is because the inflammation and damage to the skin that occurs in scarring acne affects the deeper portions of the skin rather than the constantly refreshed top layer of the skin. The changes to the deeper layers that are seen in scarring acne include a change in the amount of collagen and a transformation of the structure of the underlying tissue. Both of these changes contribute to the permanence of acne scars.

It is important to appreciate the difference between acne scars and other changes in the skin that occur as a result of acne. One of the most common effects of acne on the skin includes postinflammatory hyperpigmentation and postinflammatory hypopigmentation. These involve the changing of the color of the skin after inflammation from acne. Although anyone can experience discoloration, it is especially common in people with darker skin tones. Thankfully, unlike acne scarring, postinflammatory hyperpigmentation and hypopigmentation are temporary. While they can still take several months and up to a year to fully improve, the pigment changes do eventually go away, and the affected skin should become normalized and evenly blend into the surrounding skin.

One of the ways to tell the difference between postinflammatory hyperpigmentation or hypopigmentation and acne scarring includes assessing for changes in skin texture. Since pigment changes in the skin only affect the skin tone and not the texture of the skin, differences in elevation as compared to the surrounding skin can be a sign that acne scarring is more likely to be involved. People with acne scarring will have skin that looks pockmarked or uneven and bumpy, whereas those with postinflammatory pigment changes will still have flat, smooth skin, albeit unevenly colored.

While people with acne scarring used to have to live their lives with the condition in prior decades, the modern era has made access to effective acne scarring treatments better than ever before. In fact, most people can experience moderate to significant improvement of their acne scarring through multiple sessions of therapy, such as laser resurfacing, dermabrasion, filler, or another proven treatment.

So, while acne scarring is a permanent and troubling condition when left untreated, the ability to effectively treat and significantly improve the appearance of acne scars has changed acne scarring into a highly treatable condition. Even for people with severe acne scarring, for whom multiple treatments may be required and the skin might never be completely perfect, significant improvements in the amount of scarring can still be expected and can help to make their lesions much less visible and more bearable.

54. What treatments are available for acne scarring?

There has been an explosion in the availability of treatments for acne scarring in the past few decades. The development of powerful lasers and light therapies has made treatment for acne scarring more attainable for a broader portion of society. In addition, an improved understanding of how the skin reacts to dermabrasion, chemical peels, microneedling, and filler has allowed the cosmetic and medical community to more effectively use these therapies in the treatment of acne scars.

The specific treatment that will be most effective for an acne scar depends on the specific type of scarring that has occurred. The main two categories of acne scarring include depressed scars and elevated scars. Although there are additional subtypes and nuances of acne scars, these two general categories help to best select which type of treatments will be most effective.

The best treatments for depressed acne scars, which are scars that are lower than the surrounding skin, include therapies to help stimulate the production of collagen to help raise the overlying surface and make it more even with the surrounding area. Laser resurfacing, skin needling, dermabrasion, and filler placement are the most common techniques used in this regard.

In laser resurfacing, a powerful laser is used to target the deeper layers of the skin and apply heat energy to destroy damaged areas, allowing new healing and collagen production to correct and improve the appearance of scars. While the deepest acne scars may not be able to be treated with laser resurfacing, resurfacing lasers are able to reach and treat mild to moderate acne scarring rather effectively. Laser resurfacing can be uncomfortable, but the use of numbing agents helps to make it more comfortable. The results of the treatment include improved appearance of scars, improved skin tone and texture, and a reduction in facial lines and wrinkles.

In microneedling and dermabrasion, mechanical tools are used to cause microdamage to the underlying layers of the skin to prompt collagen production and skin repair with the goal of lifting the depressed scars so that they become even with the surrounding skin. In microneedling, tiny needles are used to create the microwounds that prompt skin healing, while in dermabrasion, a rough spinning surface is used. Although more treatments are typically required for dermabrasion and microneedling to show the same results as laser resurfacing, they are usually more affordable and less uncomfortable.

Recently, the use of fillers has become increasingly popular for treating acne scarring in addition to a variety of other cosmetic purposes, including lip enhancement and skin rejuvenation. Hyaluronic acid, collagen, and other filler materials can be injected into the skin underneath depressed scars to fill the underlying space and elevate the skin to be more even in texture with surrounding skin. While using fillers can be a highly effective treatment for acne scars, the results are temporary and last only between one to five years. Therefore, repeat treatment is needed to maintain the improvements in skin appearance.

As opposed to depressed scars, elevated scars are treated with a variety of techniques aimed at reducing the amount of underlying connective tissue to lower the scarred area to be flush with the surrounding skin. The most popular treatments for elevated scars include medical injections, microneedling, and minor surgical revision.

The most common injectable medicine for elevated acne scarring involves steroid medications that help to thin and soften the scarred area. The effects of steroid injection continue to work on the skin for days to weeks following an injection, and they can result in significant improvements in the appearance of elevated acne scars. However, steroids can have profound effects on the skin and lead to color changes and an increased risk of infection. In addition, many larger scars require multiple repeated treatments with steroid injections to show satisfactory improvement.

Microneedling and minor surgical revision are used similarly in elevated scars as they are in depressed scars. However, the ultimate aim of their use in elevated scars is to remove the extra damaged tissue and allow the healing process to place the correct amount of collagen in the new space. Therefore, they are effective tools that can be used in both elevated and depressed scars with great results.

With the blossoming of options available for the treatment of acne scarring, the perception that acne scarring has to be a lifelong struggle has significantly changed. Acne scarring has become a more manageable and treatable medical condition than ever before.

❖

Case Studies

1. AIDEN SEES HIS DOCTOR ABOUT HIS ACNE

Aiden is a fifteen-year-old male who lives at home with his older brother and sister, and he is a freshman at the local public high school. Like his older brother and sister, Aiden began to have mild acne on his face when he turned thirteen years old.

For the past year or two, Aiden's acne was not much of a bother to him. He would occasionally get small acne bumps on his forehead that were not noticeable under his hair, and the bumps would usually go away on their own within a week or two. They were rarely itchy or red. He did not pay much attention to the acne bumps because they were not very frequent or uncomfortable. In addition, Aiden had been generally healthy throughout his whole life with no medical conditions or doctor's visits besides his regular yearly checkup. He had never needed to take any kind of medicine on a regular basis.

However, since turning fifteen, Aiden has noticed that his acne has been more frequent and bothersome. Instead of happening every couple of weeks, Aiden has felt that his acne appears on different parts of his face on a weekly basis. In addition, the acne bumps that he has been experiencing are much more apparent to other people because they now occur on the cheeks, chin, lower forehead, and even around his nose. Unfortunately, for the first time, Aiden has felt more self-conscious about his acne and embarrassed about what other people might think of him because of his acne.

Upon realizing that his acne is worse than before, Aiden tried to search for tips about taking care of acne on Google. He read that changing his pillowcases and showering every day might help improve acne. He attempted both of those things, but his acne has remained persistent. Now that he has not been able to alleviate his acne with the simple fixes that he read about online, Aiden wants to try medicine for treating his acne.

Aiden is covered under his parent's health insurance plan, so he approaches his parents and asks them to take him to a doctor for his acne. His parents are supportive of this because they both had acne growing up and can appreciate the impact that it might be having on Aiden. His mom calls to make an appointment for a dermatologist, but the local dermatologist does not have any available appointments for the next three months. Aiden's mom then calls his family doctor and is able to make an appointment for later that same week.

On the day of the appointment, Aiden and his mom arrive on time to the family doctor's office. They are called back into the patient examination room after waiting about fifteen minutes in the waiting area. In the examination room, a nurse comes to check on Aiden; she takes his blood pressure and asks him about his acne. About fifteen minutes later, Aiden's family doctor arrives in the examination room and examines Aiden. He asks Aiden about his symptoms and how long they have been bothering him, and he takes a thorough history and does a physical exam. After the exam, Aiden's doctor tells him that he has a classic form of acne that should respond very well to medications. He recommends a face wash that has a chemical called benzoyl peroxide in it as well as a gel with the chemical adapalene (also known as Differin gel). He explains that both of these products are available over the counter, which means that Aiden does not need a prescription to purchase them.

Aiden's family doctor then explains how Aiden should use these medications. He explains that Aiden should gently wash his face every morning with the benzoyl peroxide face wash and to see how his skin responds to this routine after one week. If Aiden's skin is not irritated, he can then add the adapalene gel to his daily routine as well. He warns Aiden that the adapalene can be very irritating to the skin, so he recommends using it once every other day for a week or two and then increasing the frequency to every day once his skin gets used to the medication. He also warns that adapalene can cause sunburns by making the skin sensitive to sunlight, so he recommends putting the adapalene on the skin before bedtime and making sure to use sunscreen whenever going out during the daytime.

Aiden asks his family doctor how long it usually takes for acne to improve and whether these medications will completely cure his acne.

The family doctor answers that Aiden might see his acne get worse after starting the medications, but after four to six weeks of regularly using acne medications, most acne tends to improve significantly. He clarifies that there is no perfect cure for acne and that Aiden may still experience some acne bumps from time to time, but, overall, his acne should be much better controlled while using the medications.

Aiden thanks his doctor for his time and returns home excited to start his new skin-care routine for treating his acne. He experiences a flare of his acne when starting the medications, just like his doctor had mentioned, but over the course of approximately six weeks, Aiden sees his acne improve significantly. He sometimes experiences small acne bumps on the sides of his forehead, but the rest of his face has cleared up a lot. He feels much more confident and less bothered by the appearance of his skin, and his parents agree that his acne has improved. He continues to use the benzoyl peroxide wash every morning and the adapalene gel every evening to prevent more acne from appearing, and he is comfortable with this daily routine.

Analysis

Aiden's story is one of the most common experiences for adolescents and teenagers who suffer from acne. Almost all people experience acne at some point during their teenage years. For some of these people, the acne is mild enough that it does not bother them, but for many others, the acne is bothersome enough that it prompts them to seek medical treatment.

For most of these people, a simple regimen of benzoyl peroxide or other medical face wash in addition to adapalene, tretinoin, or another retinoid medication will be extremely effective at managing acne. The most important factors when using this regimen is to start slow, with just the face wash, to minimize skin irritation and build up to a daily routine with both medications over the span of a week or two. In addition, some people can get disheartened when they do not immediately see an improvement of their acne; even with the perfect treatment regimen, acne can take four to six weeks to clear up, so patience and persistence are crucial.

Thankfully, Aiden's acne was very responsive to first-line treatments and showed a significant improvement. Therefore, he did not need to seek the care of a dermatology specialist. For people whose acne does not get better or who suffer from acne with red bumps or scarring, getting medical treatment from a dermatology specialist is often the only way to get control of their acne bumps.

2. JASMINE GETS TREATMENT FOR
HER STUBBORN DARK SPOTS

Jasmine is an eighteen-year-old African American female who recently started college at the University of Buffalo. She has had mild to moderate acne throughout her teenage years, which she has been treating with a daily benzoyl peroxide face wash and a nightly retinoid cream. This has worked fairly well for her, and her acne is usually under great control.

Unfortunately, since Jasmine has started college, she has noticed more outbreaks of her acne than she remembers experiencing before. She believes that her acne tends to flare up during stressful exam weeks and whenever she has a large school assignment due. When she experiences these acne flares, she continues to use her benzoyl peroxide face wash and retinoid cream every day, which helps to make the acne flare quiet down and go away within a week.

However, Jasmine has noticed that after her acne outbreaks get better, the color of the skin on her face looks blotchier than before. In fact, the areas of the skin that the acne affected usually look darker than the surrounding skin. This change is very noticeable to Jasmine, who feels uncomfortable and embarrassed.

Although Jasmine has been able to cover up the dark spots with the use of foundation and other makeup products, she brings up the topic with her roommate, Amelia, who has also had acne throughout the past several years. Amelia shares that she also experiences dark spots after acne outbreaks and states that she has spoken with her dermatologist about this issue in the past. In addition to continuing to use retinoid creams and sunscreen, Amelia's dermatologist recommended that she use a cream with azelaic acid on the dark spots to help lighten them.

Jasmine is interested by the idea of using a skin-care product to lighten her dark spots, so she goes to her local skin-care store to search for a cream with azelaic acid. She finds a lightening cream spot treatment that has the ingredient, and she begins to use it. Although she does not see an immediate change, she does begin to notice her dark spots improving in color over the course of approximately one month. She shares this news with Amelia, who is happy that Jasmine has seen improvement in her dark spots with the treatment.

However, a week later, Jasmine spends most of a three-day-weekend outside in the sunlight because of a big football weekend. During this time in the sun, Jasmine forgets to use her sunscreen regularly and gets a lot of sun exposure on the skin of her face, neck, and arms. After the weekend is over, she notices that her dark spots are worse than ever before. She shares this with Amelia, who asks whether Jasmine remembered to continue using her sunscreen. Jasmine says that she forgot to wear her sunscreen over the weekend and vows to not forget to wear her sunscreen again.

Jasmine's dark spots are worse than before, they continue to improve with the regular use of her skin-care products and sunscreen. A few months later, Jasmine returns home for winter break and makes an appointment with her dermatologist, Dr. Kay. When speaking with Dr. Kay, Jasmine mentions her dark spots and seeks Dr. Kay's advice regarding them. Dr. Kay explains how the dark spots that are seen after acne outbreaks are a result of the inflammation that occurs during acne flares. Inflammation in the skin from acne causes melanocytes to increase production of melanin, which is the major pigment that gives skin its color. This increased production of melanin by melanocytes causes the skin to become dark in spots where acne used to be, causing the skin to appear splotchy and uneven.

Dr. Kay supports Jasmine's use of lightening treatments with azelaic acid and reinforces the importance of wearing sunscreen and continuing to use her acne treatments. In addition, Dr. Kay says that if any dark spots are particularly bothersome and do not go away with treatments, her office would be able to treat the spots with the use of a special dermatology laser. Jasmine is appreciative of Dr. Kay's advice and returns home, content that she has been doing the right things to treat her acne and her dark spots.

Analysis

The dark spots that Jasmine is experiencing after her acne outbreaks are called postinflammatory hyperpigmentation by dermatologists. The term *postinflammatory* refers to the fact that the dark spots happen after inflammation, and *hyperpigmentation* refers to the dark spots being caused by an extra amount of pigment in the skin. While postinflammatory hyperpigmentation can happen to anyone who experiences inflammation in the skin, it is most commonly seen in people who have darker skin tones.

While postinflammatory hyperpigmentation goes away on its own, this process can take several months or up to a year without the use of medications. Therefore, people commonly use retinoids, lightening creams, and even laser treatments to help postinflammatory hyperpigmentation improve more rapidly. Importantly, sun exposure causes the skin to darken, which can make dark spots and the surrounding skin even more uneven. This is why Jasmine experienced the skin changes that she noticed after spending a weekend in the sun without sunscreen, and this is why dermatologists recommend the persistent use of sunscreen to avoid uneven skin tanning in people with postinflammatory hyperpigmentation.

Although postinflammatory hyperpigmentation is not a dangerous or harmful condition, it can cause a lot of concern, especially when it happens in visible areas of the skin, such as the face. This can lead to embarrassment and lowered self-confidence. Although there is no treatment that can immediately fix postinflammatory hyperpigmentation, there are thankfully many options to help it improve more quickly and allow the skin to regain its even color more rapidly.

3. OLIVIA OVERCOMES HER SEVERE ACNE

Olivia is a sixteen-year-old female high school student. She has an older brother and sister who both suffered from moderate acne during their teenage years. Olivia has suffered from acne for a couple of years, but she has noticed that her acne has gotten worse over the past few months. While many of Olivia's friends have acne as well, she has noticed that her acne tends to be more red and painful. In fact, over the past month, Olivia has noticed that most of her face is covered with acne bumps, and she believes that her acne is the worst out of all of her friends.

Olivia's acne has caused a lot of embarrassment, and she did not feel comfortable about going to her school's homecoming dance. Olivia believes that she has become more depressed and anxious because of the severity of her acne, and she shares these concerns with her sister. Her sister encourages Olivia to let her parents know so that they can get her help for her acne. When Olivia shares her concerns with her parents, they are supportive and call their family physician, Dr. Matthews, to schedule a visit for Olivia regarding treatment for her acne.

Olivia is able to meet with Dr. Matthews for an appointment the following afternoon, and she shares her concerns regarding her acne with him. Dr. Matthews examines her face and asks her multiple questions regarding her acne, including assessing how long it has been occurring, what treatments she has been using, and what changes she has recently noticed with it. After his questions and examination, Dr. Matthews speaks with Olivia and shares that he is concerned regarding her acne because of how severe it is. He states that severe acne is best treated by a dermatologist who specializes in treating skin conditions. He recommends meeting with a dermatologist because severe acne can result in permanent scarring if it is not treated quickly and effectively. Dr. Matthews makes a referral for a local dermatologist, and Olivia is able to make an appointment with the dermatologist within the week.

Olivia attends her appointment with the dermatologist, who diagnoses her with a severe form of acne known as nodulocystic acne. The dermatologist explains that Olivia's acne is more severe than most people's, and he explains that this might be due to a variety of factors, including genetics and the body's response to bacteria that live on the skin. He shows her that her acne bumps go deep into the skin, forming nodules and cysts with fluid inside of them. He explains that she will need stronger acne medications to take control of her acne quickly and prevent as much scarring as possible. He continues to say that she likely does have some scarring already, but by starting medical treatment as soon as possible, she can reduce the amount of scarring that happens.

Olivia and her parents talk about this together, and they decide to pursue medical treatment for her severe nodulocystic acne. Olivia shares this decision with her dermatologist, who recommends starting treatment with an oral medication known as isotretinoin (Accutane). He explains that this is a powerful oral medication that helps the skin become more regulated and normal. He continues on to say that this medication is safe for most people, but it can have some significant side effects, including affecting the liver. Therefore, people who start isotretinoin need to have blood work every so often to make sure that they are not having these side effects. In addition, Olivia's dermatologist shares that isotretinoin can have a significant impact on babies whose mothers are on isotretinoin when they are pregnant; therefore, Olivia will need to be on two forms of birth control and have a negative pregnancy test before starting the medicine. This will be tracked by a system called iPLEDGE to protect Olivia from unexpected pregnancy while on the medication.

Olivia, with the support of her parents, agrees to begin treatment for her severe nodulocystic acne with isotretinoin. After starting oral birth control and agreeing to use condoms if she is sexually active, Olivia has blood work drawn that confirms she is not pregnant. She begins to take isotretinoin, and although her skin is rougher and drier than usual at first, she slowly begins to see her acne improve over the course of several months. At approximately six months, she is ecstatic to see that her acne has significantly improved. Although she does have some scarring on her cheeks, she is grateful that she started isotretinoin, which prevented more scars from forming. Her confidence in her appearance increases, and she believes that she is less depressed and anxious overall.

Analysis

For most people with mild to moderate acne, beginning treatment with topical medications is a reasonable place to start. However, for people with moderate to severe acne, or acne that has nodules and cysts, there is a need for quick and effective treatment of acne by a dermatologist as soon as possible. This is because people with these more severe forms of acne are more prone to permanent scarring. Although this scarring can sometimes be improved by lasers and cosmetic procedures, it is best to effectively treat acne and prevent scars from forming in the first place. This is why Olivia was referred to a dermatologist by her family physician and why she was started on isotretinoin, which is one of the most powerful and effective medications available for treating acne.

While isotretinoin does have some significant side effects, including affecting the liver and causing potential harm to developing fetuses, regular blood work and the iPLEDGE program reduce the risk of these side effects occurring. Isotretinoin is usually started at a lower dose for several weeks to assess the response of the skin and then increased to a maintenance dose that is given over the course of several months. Most people see a dramatic improvement in their acne after being treated with isotretinoin. However, the need for regular monitoring for all people on the medication and the use of multiple forms of birth control for people who can become pregnant means that isotretinoin is usually reserved for more severe forms of acne that require stronger medications to control.

4. KALIL GETS HELP FOR HER HORMONAL ACNE

Kalil is a twenty-four-year-old female who works as a paralegal at a local law firm. She had mild to moderate acne throughout her teenage years, but she was able to keep good control of her symptoms with a basic acne care regimen that included benzoyl peroxide and a retinoid cream. In fact, Kalil's acne had been mostly resolved since graduating from college at age twenty-one.

Unfortunately, since starting her job as a paralegal approximately one year ago, Kalil has noticed that her acne has returned. During this past year, Kalil has found her job stressful because of the amount of work she is assigned and the long hours that she is at the office. She has also noticed that she has gained about forty pounds since beginning to work as a paralegal, which she blames on the long hours and frequently ordering food from restaurants more since she does not have time to cook. She wonders whether her recent stress and weight gain are associated with her acne, so she calls a local dermatologist and schedules an appointment for a new patient evaluation. She is able to get an appointment for one month later, which she attends.

At the appointment, Kalil meets with one of the resident dermatologists, Dr. Kennedy, who asks her about her acne. In addition to asking about her recent weight gain and new acne outbreaks, Dr. Kennedy asks about Kalil's menstrual cycle and whether she has noticed any changes in the regularity or duration of her period. Kalil does note that her periods have become less regular and more infrequent. In fact, she does not believe that she has had a full period in several months. Since Kalil is not sexually active, she is not concerned about being pregnant, but she does ask Dr. Kennedy why she has not had regular periods recently.

In response to Kalil's concerns, Dr. Kennedy explains that Kalil's acne resembles what dermatologists refer to as hormonal acne. When Dr. Kennedy examined Kalil's skin, he noticed that the acne was mostly along her jaw and cheeks, which are the typical areas that hormonal acne affects. This type of acne is associated with imbalances in the body's hormones, especially in young adult women. He explains that hormonal acne is often accompanied by another condition known as polycystic ovarian syndrome, also known as PCOS.

In PCOS, there can be irregular menstrual periods, hair growth in areas where hair did not grow before, and hormonal acne. While having hormonal acne does not mean that Kalil definitely has PCOS, the fact that she has noticed irregular periods and recent weight gain means that she should make an appointment with an obstetrician and gynecologist (OBGYN) to be examined and evaluated. Before ending the visit, Dr. Kennedy also offers a couple of different treatment options for Kalil's hormonal acne, including medications that influence the body's hormone levels, such as oral birth control pills and spironolactone. Kalil is interested but asks to wait until she sees an OBGYN before she makes a decision. Although she is concerned about potentially having PCOS, she is happy that she has a better understanding of why she has been experiencing the new acne and irregular periods.

A few weeks later, Kalil is able to meet with her OBGYN. At her appointment, they speak together regarding PCOS and the possibility that Kalil might be affected. Her OBGYN orders some blood work, which does indicate that Kalil likely has PCOS. Her OBGYN explains that many young women have PCOS and that this is a condition that we know a lot about. She recommends that Kalil get blood work done to evaluate for associated conditions, such as diabetes, and that she adopt lifestyle changes to manage her recent weight gain, since being overweight or obese can increase the risk of PCOS. Kalil agrees and appreciates the guidance and then asks about her hormonal acne and whether it would be a good idea to start hormonal medications.

Her OBGYN explains that many people with PCOS suffer from hormonal acne and irregular periods and that using oral birth control pills or medications such as spironolactone that block testosterone are safe and effective approaches. Kalil agrees with this and decides to begin treatment with an oral birth control pill. Over the following months, she notes some improvement of her acne, and she notices that her menstrual cycle is regular again. She also implements lifestyle changes to manage her weight and is able to lose one pound a week with the help of a dietitian.

Analysis

Hormonal acne is a common form of acne that primarily affects women. It often presents with acne along the jaw and cheeks, and it can be associated with the menstrual cycle. It is thought to be a result of imbalances in the body's hormones, and it can be associated with conditions such as PCOS.

While the exact cause of PCOS is unclear, increased levels of insulin and testosterone are thought to be contributing factors. It is thought that being overweight or obese, significant stress, and a variety of conditions such as diabetes and sleep apnea are all risk factors for developing PCOS. The development of hormonal acne is important because it can be one of the first signs that someone is experiencing PCOS.

In addition, hormonal acne is treated with the same medications as regular acne, such as benzoyl peroxide and retinoids, and it often requires additional medications that target the hormone imbalance to fully improve. These medications can include oral birth control pills, which regulate the body's hormone balances, as well as spironolactone, which reduces the activity of testosterone in the body. When followed correctly, acne medication regimens targeted at hormonal acne can result in significant improvement within a couple of months.

5. PATRICK TREATS HIS SCARS WITH LASER THERAPY

Patrick is a twenty-seven-year-old male college student who is completing his master's degree in computer science at the local university. Patrick is married and has two young children and a pet dog. He has been very happy and has felt fulfilled in his life.

When Patrick was a teenager in high school and undergraduate college, he suffered from severe acne. Although he was interested in getting treatment for his acne, he felt embarrassed to visit a dermatologist or speak to a doctor about his concerns. Therefore, he did not use any medications for his acne. Although his acne eventually improved and went away in his midtwenties, the skin on his face was permanently affected by many small scars.

Patrick was not overly concerned about his physical appearance, but he did sometimes linger when looking at his face in the mirror. He occasionally wondered about getting treatment from a dermatologist for his scars, but he was not sure how to go about finding a dermatologist that would treat him.

One evening, Patrick mentioned his concerns to his wife, whose face lit up. She had been to a cosmetic dermatologist several years past, and she recommended that he make an appointment, which he did the next morning. Although the closest appointment was several months away, Patrick was excited to be able to get care for the scars that he was worried would affect him for his whole life.

When the appointment finally came around, Patrick visited the cosmetic dermatologist's office, and he was brought into one of the patient examination rooms. When the dermatologist eventually entered the room, she introduced herself as Dr. Naz and asked Patrick about his acne. After completing her examination and taking his medical history, she began to make some recommendations and educate him about his acne.

Dr. Naz informed Patrick that the acne that he suffered from as a teenager had permanently affected the surface of his skin and the connective tissue that was underneath the skin. She shared that many people with untreated acne develop such scarring because the inflammation causes the skin to become lower than the surrounding skin, leaving a pockmarked appearance. She shared that although those marks do not heal on their own, there are medical and cosmetic treatments available to help improve scarring from acne.

Dr. Naz shared with Patrick the concept of laser resurfacing for treating his acne scars. As Patrick understood it, the general process was that Dr. Naz would use a powerful laser to break apart the scar tissue near the surface of the skin. This would also stimulate the production of collagen and the reorganization of the cells and connective tissue near the skin. Ultimately, the end result would be a more even texture to the skin and an improvement in the appearance of the acne scars.

Patrick asked Dr. Naz whether the procedure would hurt and how many times he would have to undergo laser resurfacing to see an effect on his acne. She explained that the laser resurfacing is uncomfortable, but numbing gels can be used to help reduce the discomfort associated with the treatment. She continued to explain that while one treatment would still benefit his skin, she recommended about three or four treatments to get the maximum effect.

Patrick was appreciative to Dr. Naz for explaining the idea of laser resurfacing and answering his questions, and he asked Dr. Naz for time to speak with his wife about the topic. Dr. Naz thanked him for visiting her and said that if he chose to pursue laser resurfacing, she would be happy to take care of him.

That evening, Patrick spoke with his wife regarding the plan to start laser resurfacing. Although it was expensive by their standards, they both agreed that treating his acne scars would result in an improvement in Patrick's happiness and well-being. Therefore, Patrick called Dr. Naz's office and scheduled his course of laser resurfacing therapy.

Over the next few months, Patrick underwent three laser resurfacing treatments. Although the procedure was uncomfortable and left his skin feeling sore afterward, the numbing treatments beforehand helped to make it more bearable. After his last resurfacing session, Patrick was asked to follow up within three months to evaluate how he had responded to the course of treatment. By the time that he attended the follow-up appointment, Patrick noted significant improvement in his acne scars. Rather than being pockmarked, the skin of his face had become much more even and clear. While it was possible to tell some minor texture changes in the skin, it was much less obvious that he had suffered from acne as a younger man. Patrick thanked Dr. Naz for the treatment, and he shared with her that his acne scars had caused him a lot of stress and embarrassment throughout his life and that he was extremely grateful for her care.

Analysis

One of the most significant side effects of acne is the presence of acne scarring, which is a permanent change in the skin. Unfortunately, acne scarring can cause just as much psychological and emotional distress as acne itself. Although acne scarring was largely untreatable several decades ago, the development of new treatments for acne scars has allowed dermatologists and other cosmetic professionals to effectively treat the condition.

While there are a variety of treatments for acne scars, the underlying principle is that a medication or procedure will help to make the skin more even and break up scar issue that has formed. In the case of acne scars that are depressed, meaning lower than the surrounding skin, treatments focus on stimulating the production of new collagen, which can help to elevate the depressed scar. Laser resurfacing treatments are a very popular method of treating acne scars, but skin needling, dermabrasion, and even skin fillers can be effective as well.

Although no treatment can completely and perfectly cure acne scars, most people can significantly reduce the visibility and severity of their acne scars with treatment. For people with acne scars, these treatments can be life changing by improving self-esteem and reducing embarrassment, self-consciousness, and even anxiety or depression.

Glossary

Acne fulminans: A sudden and severe flare of acne that can cause a flu-like experience, including aching muscles and joints, significant redness all over, and a fever with chills and sweating.

Acne rosacea: The medical term for rosacea, which is a skin condition that causes blushing or redness of the skin of the face as well as small visible blood vessels and occasionally little red spots that can mimic classic acne.

Acne vulgaris: The medical term for classic acne, which is derived from Latin. It is associated with blackheads, whiteheads, pimples, nodules, and cysts and is thought to occur as a result of the interaction between skin pores, natural oils, bacteria, hormones, and inflammation.

Androgens: The group of hormones that is responsible for male characteristics in the body, including deeper voice, increased muscle mass, and genital development. Androgens have been shown to play an important role in contributing to the development of acne by stimulating the oil-producing glands of the skin.

Benzoyl peroxide: The most commonly recommended face wash that is one of the cornerstones of treating all forms of acne. It is similar in function to salicylic acid and other cleansers that are newly available on the market.

Comedones: The medical term for the blocked skin pore that causes acne. Blackheads and whiteheads are both different forms of comedones, and pimples are comedones that have become filled with inflammation. Medications that break apart clogged skin pores to help improve acne are known as comedolytics.

Fitzpatrick scale: The most commonly used system for describing skin tone based on the way that skin responds to sunlight, ranging from a Fitzpatrick type I that is so fair that it only ever burns in response to sunlight up to a Fitzpatrick type VII that never burns and only tans.

Glycemic index: A measure of how quickly a food increases the level of sugar in the bloodstream, which has been shown to determine how likely a food might cause an acne flare. High glycemic index foods, such as candy, increase the level of sugar in the blood rapidly and have been shown to be associated with acne.

iPLEDGE: The federally mandated program that people are required to register with before starting medical therapy with isotretinoin (Accutane). As part of the iPLEDGE program, people taking isotretinoin are required to get regular blood work, and people who are able to become pregnant are required to use multiple forms of contraception and to take regular pregnancy tests as well.

Isotretinoin: Also known by the brand name, Accutane. This is the most commonly prescribed oral retinoid for treating acne, and it is extremely effective in improving the appearance of skin over the course of several months. However, it does have significant side effects that require close monitoring by a physician.

Melanocytes: The cells of the body that are responsible for creating and distributing the pigment that gives skin, hair, and nails their color.

Nodulocystic acne: A form of acne where there is significant inflammation that causes deep bumps within the skin, known as nodules, and pockets of pus-filled fluid, known as cysts. This form of acne is highly scarring due to the increased levels of inflammation.

Noncomedogenic: A skin-care product that is specially designed to not block skin pores or worsen acne.

Over the counter: Medications and treatments that are available to individuals without the need for a prescription from a physician or other health-care provider.

Polycystic ovarian syndrome (PCOS): A very common metabolic condition affecting women that is associated with increased testosterone levels, irregular periods, facial and body hair, and acne.

Propionibacterium acnes: A species of bacteria that lives on the skin of the majority of people in the world that has been implicated in contributing to acne by feeding on the natural skin oils and creating chemicals that can increase inflammation in the skin.

Retinoids: A class of medications that include oral and topical medicines that share a similar structure to vitamin A and are able to significantly improve acne by controlling the behavior of skin cells through chemical and cellular pathways.

Ultraviolet (UV): A category of radiation that has a wavelength between 10 and 400 nanometers. Sunlight is a form of ultraviolet radiation that can cause skin damage when there is excessive exposure to daylight. Sunscreen and sun avoidance are effective ways of avoiding ultraviolet radiation.

Directory of Resources

BOOKS

Cho, Charlotte. *The Little Book of Skin Care: Korean Beauty Secrets for Healthy, Glowing Skin*. William Morrow, 2015.

Fu, Victoria. *Skincare Decoded: The Practical Guide to Beautiful Skin*. Weldon Owen, 2021.

Service, Katie. *The Beauty Brief: An Insider's Guide to Skincare*. Thames and Hudson, 2021.

Viera-Newton, Rio. *Let's Face It: Secrets of a Skincare Obsessive*. Voracious, 2021.

ORGANIZATIONS

Acne Care and Education Society (ACnE Society)
https://www.societyforacne.org
ACnE Society is committed to the mission of working toward fulfilling the current gaps in medical knowledge and social awareness in acne care by providing support to acne sufferers and acne researchers.

American Academy of Dermatology (AAD)
https://www.aad.org
The AAD is the largest and most influential representative dermatology group in the United States. With a membership of more than 20,500

physicians worldwide, the AAD is committed to advancing the diagnosis and treatment of skin conditions, advocating high standards in dermatology, and supporting and enhancing patient care.

American Acne and Rosacea Society (AARS)
https://acneandrosacea.org
The mission of the AARS is to serve as an educational forum for the exchange of information related to acne and rosacea, to promote research and mentoring opportunities for dermatology professionals, and to improve the care of patients who suffer from acne and rosacea.

National Institute of Arthritis and Musculoskeletal and Skin Diseases (NIAMS)
https://www.niams.nih.gov/health-topics/acne
The mission of the NIAMS is to support research into the causes, treatment, and prevention of arthritis and musculoskeletal and skin diseases; the training of basic and clinical scientists to carry out this research; and the dissemination of information on research progress in these diseases.

WEBSITES

American Academy of Dermatology acne resource center: https://www.aad.org/public/diseases/acne

Healthtalk acne overview: https://healthtalk.org/acne/overview

NeutrogenaMD acne resources: https://www.neutrogenamd.com/acne

UpToDate Acne, beyond the basics: https://www.uptodate.com/contents/acne-beyond-the-basics

Verywell Health acne guide: https://www.verywellhealth.com/acne-overview-4581760

Index

Accutane. *See* Isotretinoin
Acne: causes, 25–27; childhood,
    4, 15; chloracne, 46; classic,
    3, 5, 6–7, 14, 45; conglobata,
    13; fulminans, 13, 75, 117;
    hormonal, 4, 11, 78–80; infantile,
    15; inflammatory, 3, 10, 13;
    medicamentosa, 30–31, 44–46;
    neonatal, 4, 15; nodulocystic,
    13, 93
Acne fulminans, definition
    of, 117
Acne rosacea, definition of, 117
Adolescence, and acne,
    14–15
Alcohol, 34
Alternative therapies: acupuncture,
    85; Ayurveda, 84; honey, 84; tea
    tree oil, 84
American Academy of Dermatology
    (AAD), 63
Anatomy: blackheads, 3, 9–10, 25;
    comedones, 3, 9–10; follicles, 3,
    8–10, 15, 22, 25–27, 70; sebaceous

glands, 8, 25, 27; whiteheads, 3,
    8–10, 25
Androgens, definition of, 117

Benzoyl peroxide, 44, 59–60, 69–71,
    74–75, 78–79, 83–84, 85–86, 91,
    98; costs of, 88; definition of, 117
Body mass index (BMI), 32–33

Cognitive behavioral therapy, 99
Comedones, definition of, 118
Conditions that mimic acne, 21–23
Cosmetics: chemical peels, 82, 87,
    101; dermabrasion, 82, 87, 93, 98,
    101–102; fillers, 102; injections, 82,
    102; microdermabrasion, 82, 87, 98,
    101–102; microneedling, 101–102;
    resurfacing, 82, 98, 101
Cutibacterium acnes, 6–10, 26, 70

Depression, 51–53
Dermatologists, 62–63, 66, 67–69,
    82–83, 88, 89, 99
Diet, 35–36, 62

Epidemiology, 5–6, 14, 15–17, 19–20, 32–33, 49–53, 66–67, 88–89, 98

Fitzpatrick scale, 18, 20; definition of, 118
Food: chocolate, 37; elimination diet, 37; milk, 36–37

Genetics, 41–42
Glycemic index, 36; definition of, 118

Hormones: estrogen, 14–15, 28, 43–44; glucocorticoids, 28; insulin, 28, 36; steroids, 12, 45, 102; testosterone, 11–12, 14, 15, 25–26, 27–29, 78–80
Hygiene, 39–41, 58–60

iPLEDGE system, 75–78; definition of, 118
Isotretinoin, 21, 43, 72, 74–76, 77–78, 86, 87, 92, 109–110; definition of, 118

Keloids, 19

Lifestyle modifications, 60–62
Light therapy, 80–81, 98

Makeup, 38–39, 56–58
Medical conditions: androgen-secreting tumors, 30; Cushing syndrome, 30; folliculitis, 22; hidradenitis suppurativa, 76; keratosis pilaris, 22; polycystic ovarian syndrome, 17, 25, 29–30, 34; pyogenic arthritis, pyoderma gangrenosum, and acne syndrome, 47; rosacea, 19–20; sebaceous hyperplasia, 22; seborrheic dermatitis, 21; skin cancer, 23; synovitis-acne-pustulosis-hyperostosis-osteitis syndrome, 30, 47
Medications: adapalene, 88; antibiotics, 71–72; antihistamines, 56; benzoyl peroxide, 44, 59–60, 69–71, 79, 83–86, 88, 91, 98; isotretinoin, 21, 43–44, 72–78, 87, 89, 92; oral contraceptives, 11, 45, 75, 79–80, 83–84; retinoids, 72–74, 83–86, 91, 98; salicylic acid, 44; spironolactone, 29, 79–80
Melanocytes, 19, 94–95, 107; definition of, 118

National Suicide Prevention Hotline, 64
Nodulocystic acne, 13, 83, 93, 97, 109; definition of, 118
Noncomedogenic, 57; definition of, 119

Over-the-counter products, 65–66, 88; definition of, 119

Polycystic ovarian syndrome (PCOS), 17, 25, 29, 34, 111; definition of, 119
Post-inflammatory hyperpigmentation, 19, 94–95, 100
Pregnancy, 42–44
Propionibacterium acnes, 9; definition of, 119
Psychological impact, 6, 8, 11–12, 13, 48, 49–53, 63–64, 100–101

Retinoids, 44, 74, 75, 79, 83; definition of, 119; and treatment with acne, 72–74, 85–86
Rosacea, difference between acne and, 19–21

Scarring, 53–55, 81–82, 87, 95–102
Self-image, 49
Skincare routine, 58–60
Skin of color, 17–19, 96–97
Smoking, 34–35

SPF. *See* Sunscreen
Stress, 31–32
Sunscreen, 59, 61, 73–74, 86, 95
Support resources, 62–63
System to Manage Accutane-
    Related Teratogenicity (SMART)
    program, 77

Ultraviolet (UV), 18, 44, 60, 94;
    definition of, 119
U.S. Food and Drug Administration
    (FDA), 76
UV. *See* Ultraviolet

Weight gain, 32–34

About the Author

Shayan Waseh is a licensed resident physician specializing in the practice of dermatology at Temple University in Philadelphia, Pennsylvania. Originally from Buffalo, New York, Shayan received his bachelor's degree in biology from the University of Buffalo before going on to earn his postbaccalaureate from the University of Pennsylvania. Additionally, Shayan has worked in the public health space since completing a master's of public health at Thomas Jefferson University, where he subsequently completed his medical training. He has written extensively on various topics that include population health, telemedicine, and dermatology in a variety of textbooks, encyclopedias, and peer-reviewed research journals.